Cardiovascular Emergencies, Part I

Editors

MICHINARI HIEDA
GIOVANNI ESPOSITO

HEART FAILURE CLINICS

www.heartfailure.theclinics.com

Consulting Editor
EDUARDO BOSSONE

Founding Editor
JAGAT NARULA

April 2020 • Volume 16 • Number 2

ELSEVIER

1600 John F. Kennedy Boulevard • Suite 1800 • Philadelphia, Pennsylvania, 19103-2899

http://www.theclinics.com

HEART FAILURE CLINICS Volume 16, Number 2
April 2020 ISSN 1551-7136, ISBN-13: 978-0-323-73313-7

Editor: Stacy Eastman
Developmental Editor: Laura Fisher

Heart Failure Clinics (ISSN 1551-7136) is published quarterly by Elsevier Inc., 360 Park Avenue South, New York, NY 10010-1710. Months of publication are January, April, July, and October. Business and editorial offices: 1600 John F. Kennedy Boulevard, Suite 1800, Philadelphia, PA 19103-2899. Periodicals postage paid at New York, NY, and additional mailing offices. Subscription prices are USD 269.00 per year for US individuals, USD 534.00 per year for US institutions, USD 100.00 per year for US students and residents, USD 300.00 per year for Canadian individuals, USD 618.00 per year for Canadian institutions, USD 315.00 per year for international individuals, USD 618.00 per year for international institutions, and USD 100.00 per year for Canadian and foreign students/residents. To receive student and resident rate, orders must be accompanied by name of affiliated institution, date of term, and the *signature* of program/residency coordinator on institution letterhead. Orders will be billed at individual rate until proof of status is received. Foreign air speed delivery is included in all *Clinics* subscription prices. All prices are subject to change without notice. **POSTMASTER:** Send address changes to *Heart Failure Clinics*, Elsevier Health Sciences Division, Subscription Customer Service, 3251 Riverport Lane, Maryland Heights, MO 63043. **Customer Service: 1-800-654-2452 (US and Canada). From outside of the US and Canada, call 314-447-8871. Fax: 314-447-8029. For print support, E-mail: JournalsCustomerService-usa@elsevier.com. For online support, E-mail: JournalsOnlineSupport-usa@elsevier.com.**

Reprints. For copies of 100 or more of articles in this publication, please contact the Commercial Reprints Department, Elsevier Inc., 360 Park Avenue South, New York, NY 10010-1710. Tel.: 212-633-3874; Fax: 212-633-3820; E-mail: reprints@elsevier.com.

Heart Failure Clinics is covered in *MEDLINE/PubMed (Index Medicus).*

Contributors

CONSULTING EDITOR

EDUARDO BOSSONE, MD, PhD, FCCP, FESC, FACC
Division of Cardiology, AORN A Cardarelli Hospital, Naples, Italy

EDITORS

MICHINARI HIEDA, MD, MS, PhD
Senior Visiting Researcher, The University of Texas Southwestern Medical Center, Institute for Exercise and Environmental Medicine, Texas Health Presbyterian Hospital Dallas, Dallas, Texas, USA

GIOVANNI ESPOSITO, MD, PhD
Professor of Cardiology, University Federico II of Naples, Naples, Italy

AUTHORS

KOICHI AKASHI, MD
Department of Hematology, Oncology and Cardiovascular Medicine, Kyushu University Hospital, Fukuoka, Japan

SHUNICHI DOI, MD
Division of Cardiology, Department of Internal Medicine, St. Marianna University School of Medicine, Kawasaki, Kanagawa, Japan

MITSUHIRO FUKATA, MD, PhD
Assistant Professor, Department of Hematology, Oncology and Cardiovascular Medicine, Heart Center, Kyushu University Hospital, Fukuoka, Japan

RAKUSHUMIMARIKA HARADA, MD
Department of Internal Medicine, Texas Health Presbyterian Hospital of Dallas, Dallas, Texas, USA

ATSUSHI HAYASHI, MD
Second Department of Internal Medicine, University of Occupational and Environmental Health, School of Medicine, Fukuoka, Japan

MICHINARI HIEDA, MD, MS, PhD
Senior Visiting Researcher, The University of Texas Southwestern Medical Center, Institute for Exercise and Environmental Medicine, Texas Health Presbyterian Hospital Dallas, Dallas, Texas, USA

KEISUKE KIDA, MD, PhD
Department of Pharmacology, St. Marianna University School of Medicine, Kawasaki, Kanagawa, Japan

TAKESHI KITAI, MD, PhD
Departments of Cardiovascular Medicine and Clinical Research Support, Kobe City Medical Center General Hospital, Kobe, Japan

HITOSHI KUSABA, MD
Department of Hematology, Oncology and Cardiovascular Medicine, Kyushu University Hospital, Fukuoka, Japan

YOGAMAYA MANTHA, MD
Department of Internal Medicine, Texas Health Presbyterian Hospital of Dallas, Dallas, Texas, USA

TORU MARUYAMA, MD
Department of Hematology, Oncology and
Cardiovascular Medicine, Kyushu University
Hospital, Fukuoka, Japan

TOHRU MASUYAMA, MD, PhD
Director, JCHO Hoshigaoka Medical Center,
Hirakata, Osaka, Japan

SHOHEI MORIYAMA, MD
Department of Hematology,
Oncology and Cardiovascular
Medicine, Kyushu University Hospital,
Fukuoka, Japan

MASATAKA SUGAHARA, MD, PhD
JCHO Hoshigaoka Medical Center, Hirakata,
Osaka, Japan

TADAFUMI SUGIMOTO, MD, PhD, FESC
Department of Clinical Laboratory, Mie
University Hospital, Tsu, Japan

NORIO SUZUKI, MD, PhD
Division of Cardiology, Department of Internal
Medicine, St. Marianna University School of
Medicine Yokohama City Seibu Hospital,
Yokohama, Kanagawa, Japan

YUICHIRO TOMA, MD
Department of Cardiovascular Medicine,
Nephrology, and Neurology, Faculty of
Medicine, University of the Ryukyus, Okinawa,
Japan

ANDREW XANTHOPOULOS, MD, PhD
Department of Cardiology, University General
Hospital of Larissa, Larissa, Greece

Contents

Heart failure (HF) is a leading cause of hospitalization. Suitable pharmacologic management is critical. Distinct physical findings such as congestion and peripheral hypoperfusion need to be considered in selecting pharmacologic therapy. By applying the pretest probability and likelihood ratios of unique physical findings of HF to a Markov model, a definite posttest probability can be obtained. This article focuses on the findings of S3, jugular venous pressure, proportional pulse pressure, bendopnea, trepopnea, and various heart murmurs. Incorporating statistical precision in physical assessments, diagnoses of HF can be further refined, providing a sophisticated approach to evaluate patients hemodynamics status noninvasively.

This article reviews treatment and management of common cardiovascular emergencies in critically ill patients, focusing on acute decompensated heart failure, cardiogenic shock, pulmonary embolism, and hypertensive crisis management with inotropes, vasopressors, diuretics, and antiarrhythmic drugs. Clinicians frequently come across challenging clinical scenarios, and there is a gap between evidence-based medicine and clinical practice. Inotropic and vasopressor agents are useful in the acute setting but must be weaned off or used as a bridge for mechanical circulation support devices. Clinicians should aim to lower complications by choosing medications with respect to comorbidities and close the gap between evidence-based medicine and clinical practice.

The emergency room is a principal entrance for the initial management of patients with acute heart failure. Echocardiography may be performed by cardiologists and noncardiologists in the emergency room. Echocardiographic studies require effective technical skills and precise diagnostic knowledge. This article contributes to physicians in the emergency room, general practitioners in training, and medical staff who engage in emergency medicine. This article emphasized the role of echocardiography in light of pathophysiology of acute heart failure in the emergency room and refining the clinical workflow by integrating conventional and innovative knowledge for the initial management of acute heart failure.

Cardiogenic shock (CS) is the most serious complication of acute myocardial infarction (AMI). The practice of early revascularization by percutaneous coronary intervention, and advances in pharmacotherapy have reduced the rate of complications of CS. However, when CS is combined with AMI, mortality from AMI is still high, and many clinicians are wondering how to treat CS with AMI. In recent years, mechanical circulatory support (MCS) devices have improved the clinical outcome in AMI patients with CS. For best outcome, treatment of AMI with CS should always consider treatments that improve the prognosis of the patients.

Acute decompensated heart failure (ADHF) requires immediate treatments because it impairs perfusion to systemic organs and their function. Half of all patients with ADHF are diagnosed with heart failure with reduced left ventricular ejection fraction (HFrEF). The initial goal of management for ADHF is to stabilize hemodynamic status. Pulmonary edema is treated with vasodilators or diuretics. Inhibitors of the renin-angiotensin-aldosterone system and β-blockers should be started and/or increased to meet the maximum dose, ideally the target dose, that the patient can tolerate as a treatment of HFrEF. Patients with severe circulatory failure need inotropic drugs or mechanical circulatory support.

There are few treatment options for acute decompensated heart failure patients with preserved ejection fraction, but an increasing number of patients with heart failure with preserved ejection fraction. A deeper understanding of the cause, diagnosis, and prognosis of heart failure with preserved ejection fraction may be informative for clinical practice or clinical decision making and therapeutic investigation in the acute care setting.

Acute mitral regurgitation is an uncommon, challenging disease that requires emergent care and proper management. To evaluate its etiology, echocardiography is essential. However, echocardiography findings in these patients are often different from that of chronic mitral regurgitation owing to the acute elevation of left atrial and pulmonary artery pressure derived from the small left ventricle and atrium with low compliance. Although surgical correction is usually required owing to the hemodynamic instability, many patients are considered to be at high surgical risk. Transcatheter mitral valve repair using MitraClip (Abbott Vascular, Santa Clara, CA) may be a solution as a bail-out therapy.

Cardiogenic shock (CS) is a life-threatening condition characterized by end-organ hypoperfusion and hypoxia primarily due to cardiac dysfunction and low cardiac output. Unfortunately, the mortality and morbidity associated with CS have remained high despite notable advances in heart failure management. Treatment should be carefully guided by hemodynamics assessment. Although inotropes, vasopressors, mechanical circulatory support, and catheter intervention for critical valve lesion are not always recommended, they are helpful in selected patients. Early diagnosis, accurate hemodynamic assessment, and prompt therapeutic intervention are crucial in the management of acute decompensated heart failure with CS.

Several cancer treatments cause cardiotoxicity that can lead to heart failure, coronary artery disease, arrhythmia, and pericardial disease. In this review, representative cases of heart failure following cardiotoxicity caused by trastuzumab, anthracycline, and hematopoietic stem cell transplantation are described with case notes. Additionally, other important points regarding cardiotoxicity related to heart failure are reported. During and after potentially cardiotoxic therapy, periodic cardiac examinations are recommended to detect any cardiovascular disorders; these are ameliorated if appropriately diagnosed at an earlier stage. It is important for cardiologists and oncologists to understand the pathophysiology of representative cardiovascular disease cases following cancer treatment.

The heart failure (HF) guidelines recommend palliative care; however, it can often be difficult to determine the timing of palliative care referral. Because HF with fluid retention and low-cardiac output may trigger several unpleasant symptoms, continuous HF treatment is required to alleviate these symptoms in advanced HF. The patients with HF often suffer from total pain; therefore, the support from a multidisciplinary team plays a crucial role to improve quality of life of the patients and their families not only in the terminal phase but also from the early stage.

HEART FAILURE CLINICS

SERIES OF RELATED INTEREST

Cardiology Clinics
http://www.cardiology.theclinics.com/
Cardiac Electrophysiology Clinics
https://www.cardiacep.theclinics.com/
Interventional Cardiology Clinics
https://www.interventional.theclinics.com/

THE CLINICS ARE AVAILABLE ONLINE!
Access your subscription at:
www.theclinics.com

Preface

The Latest Clinical Understandings and Theory of the Cardiovascular Systems for Cardiovascular Emergencies and Their Management

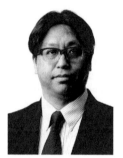

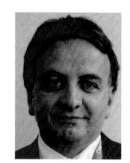

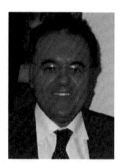

Michinari Hieda, MD, MS, PhD   Giovanni Esposito, MD, PhD   Eduardo Bossone, MD, PhD, FCCP, FESC, FACC

Editors

Cardiovascular emergencies (CE) are potentially lethal in patients admitted to emergency departments.[1,2] These conditions are remarkable for their sudden onset and often require quick differential diagnosis followed by rapid treatment interventions. For such a purpose, the clinical accurate understandings of the cardiovascular system adaptations during CE and its pathophysiology are mandatory.

Even in the accumulated evidence-based medicine (EBM) era, approximately 1.5 million cases of acute myocardial infarction (AMI) occur annually in the United States[3]; the yearly incidence rate is approximately 600 cases per 100,000 people. AMI remains the most common cause of heart failure (HF). HF is a major cause of late morbidity and mortality after AMI. Despite the establishment of standard therapy, HF remains a devastating disease that affects 6.5 million Americans $\geq$20 years of age.[3] End-stage advanced HF is associated with dramatic reductions in quality of life and a very high mortality ($\geq$80% at 5 years)[4] and thus requires special therapeutic interventions.[5] Those diseases are leading causes of hospitalizations given their high mortality.

Based on this, we here highlighted the physical examination protocols, imaging tools, and therapeutic interventions implemented in the emergency clinical scenario in patients with AMI, HF (with reduced ejection fraction and with preserved ejection fraction), acute mitral regurgitation with mitral clip intervention, and cardiogenic shock. In addition, as oncocardiology has become a recent exploding field, we deemed it relevant to add an article related to oncocardiology since the number of patients with cancer and cancer survivors with cardiovascular diseases is likely to increase in the future. Related to this, another important topic covered in this issue is palliative care in patients with advanced HF.

We prepared this issue, "Cardiovascular Emergencies, Part I," to enhance the clinical, theoretic, and rational knowledge for decision making with EBM. We weighed why clinical decisions with EBM were made and why certain therapeutic approaches were taken. Where EBM is not available, all authors attempted to present rational clinical thinking and expert consensus opinions based on their extensive clinical experience.

We are confident that the clinical information presented in this issue provides the readers with a certain framework for the understanding of the

Heart Failure Clin 16 (2020) ix–x
https://doi.org/10.1016/j.hfc.2020.01.001
1551-7136/20/© 2020 Published by Elsevier Inc.

heartfailure.theclinics.com

cardiovascular systems in CE and therapeutic strategies for CE and their management.

Finally, we would like to express our sincere gratitude to our colleagues who helped prepare this *Heart Failure Clinics* issue, including all the colleagues at University of Texas Southwestern Medical Center and University Federico II of Naples, for providing valuable suggestions, and the Elsevier team, Stacy Eastman, Laura Fisher, Vignesh Viswanathan, and Reni Thomas, for their precious editorial and production work.

Michinari Hieda, MD, MS, PhD
University of Texas
Southwestern Medical Center
Institute for Exercise and Environmental Medicine
Texas Health Presbyterian Hospital Dallas
Dallas, TX 75231, USA

Giovanni Esposito, MD, PhD
University Federico II of Naples
Via Pansini 5
80131, Naples, Italy

Eduardo Bossone, MD, PhD, FCCP, FESC, FACC
Division of Cardiology
AORN A Cardarelli Hospital
Via A. Cardarelli 9
Naples 80131, Italy

E-mail addresses:
MichinariHieda@Texashealth.org (M. Hieda)
hieda.michinari.0119@gmail.com (M. Hieda)
espogiov@unina.it (G. Esposito)
ebossone@hotmail.com (E. Bossone)

REFERENCES

1. Ibanez B, James S, Agewall S, et al. 2017 ESC guidelines for the management of acute myocardial infarction in patients presenting with ST-segment elevation: the Task Force for the management of acute myocardial infarction in patients presenting with ST-segment elevation of the European Society of Cardiology (ESC). Eur Heart J 2017;39(2):119–77.
2. Yancy CW, Jessup M, Bozkurt B, et al. 2017 ACC/AHA/HFSA focused update of the 2013 ACCF/AHA Guideline for the Management of Heart Failure: a report of the American College of Cardiology/American Heart Association Task Force on Clinical Practice Guidelines and the Heart Failure Society of America. Circulation 2017; 136(6):e137–61.
3. Benjamin EJ, Blaha MJ, Chiuve SE, et al. Heart Disease and Stroke Statistics—2017 update: a report from the American Heart Association. Circulation 2017;135(10):e146–603.
4. Friedrich EB, Böhm M. Management of end stage heart failure. Heart 2007;93(5):626–31.
5. Cleland JG, Gemmell I, Khand A, et al. Is the prognosis of heart failure improving? Eur J Heart Fail 1999;1(3):229–41.

Back to Basics
Key Physical Examinations and Theories in Patients with Heart Failure

Rakushumimarika Harada, MD[a], Yogamaya Mantha, MD[a],
Michinari Hieda, MD, MS, PhD[b],*

KEYWORDS

- Heart failure • Physical examinations • Nohria-Stevenson classification • Clinical scenarios
- Likelihood ratio • odds • Markov process • heart murmur

KEY POINTS

- Killip, Forrester, Nohria-Stevenon classification, and Clinical Scenarios are useful heart failure (HF) classifications to guide initial pharmacologic therapy and assess a patient's mortality at the time of physical examination.
- By multiplying pretest probability and several likelihood ratios, an estimated posttest probability with a higher precision for each individual patient can be obtained.
- The presence of S3, elevated jugular venous pressure (JVP), proportional pulse pressure, bendopnea, trepopnea, and other physical examination findings that are unique to HF will be helpful in assessing disease severity and hemodynamic status of a patient in relation to HF.
- As valvular diseases can affect prognosis and outcome of HF, differentiation of various types of cardiac murmurs with or without maneuvers to enhance the quality of auscultation is a valuable skill for all examiners.
- Detailed JVP changes during the cardiac cycle in association with right atrium (RA) and right ventricle (RV) pressure changes can provide insights on heart failure with either valvular or nonvalvular disease.

BACKGROUND

Heart failure (HF) is one of the most common reasons for hospitalizations. Indeed, 20% of hospitalizations of adults over 65 years are secondary to HF.[1] Acute onset HF itself has a high mortality. However, having recurrent episodes of HF can also further worsen its prognosis.[2] Hence, appropriate management and diagnosis becomes important to avoid recurrent admissions related to HF.

Medicine has been drastically transformed as technologies and laboratory testing methods have advanced over the years. Contrary to celebrations of the advancement in medical technologies, the essence of obtaining history and physical examination has been often forgotten.[3] In fact, limited

Sources of Funding: Dr. Hieda was supported by the American Heart Association Strategically Focused Research Network (14SFRN20600009-03). Dr. Hieda was also supported by American Heart Association post-doctoral fellowship grant (18POST33960092) and the Harry S. Moss Heart Trust.
a Department of Internal Medicine, Texas Health Presbyterian Hospital of Dallas, 8200 Walnut Hill Lane, Dallas, TX, 75231, USA; b Institute for Exercise and Environmental Medicine, Texas Health Presbyterian Hospital Dallas, University of Texas Southwestern Medical Center, 7232 Greenville Avenue, Dallas, TX 75231, USA
* Corresponding author.
E-mail address: michinarihieda@texashealth.org

Heart Failure Clin 16 (2020) 139–151
https://doi.org/10.1016/j.hfc.2019.12.001
1551-7136/20/© 2019 Elsevier Inc. All rights reserved.

history or physical examinations can cloud the diagnosis despite having proper images or laboratory tests. By acquiring clear history on a patient's illness and performing accurate physical examinations with high pretest probability, one can reach a correct diagnosis with higher posttest probability. This review revisits the importance of physical examinations with emphasis on pretest probability in HF encountered in the emergency room (ER) and intensive care unit/coronary care unit.

Obtaining a precise history before performing physical examination remains a fundamental step to correct diagnosis. The most common findings are paroxysmal nocturnal dyspnea, orthopnea, and dyspnea on exertion. Bilateral leg edema, abdominal swelling/discomfort, and weight gain are also commonly noted in these patients. Besides symptoms, known diagnosis of hypertension, valvular diseases, or coronary artery diseases are equally important information because these patients can present with HF in 50% to 70% of cases.[4–6] In fact, the Framingham Heart Study has shown that the incidence of HF with a history of myocardial infarction or hypertension can worsen the prognosis of survival.[6] Understanding symptoms and risk factors are crucial for us to provide appropriate medical management as there are many causes that can lead to HF. Besides carefully monitoring patient weight changes, brain natriuretic peptide levels, and chest radiograph or echocardiogram findings, incorporating characterization based on the Killip classification and Forrester classification, the Nohria-Stevenson classification, and the Clinical Scenarios at ER visit and discharge should be essential in HF diagnosis and managements.

PROGNOSTIC CLASSIFICATION
Killip Classification and Forrester Classification

The Killip classification is based on evaluation of the mortality among patients who have had acute myocardial infarction and developed acute HF. The association between hospital mortality and patients' clinical symptoms were studied by looking for absence of congestion (class I), or presence of S3/rales (class II), acute pulmonary edema (class III), and cardiogenic shock (class IV) (**Table 1**).[7] Forrester and colleagues[8] developed a characterization of HF in patients with acute myocardial infarction from both hemodynamics and clinical perspectives. Pulmonary capillary wedge pressure (PCWP) and cardiac index (CI) were measured to evaluate cardiac function, whereas pulmonary congestion (ie, presence of posttussive rales, radiographic evidence of congestion) and peripheral perfusion (ie, diminished skin perfusion, oliguria with arterial hypoperfusion) were observed clinically (**Table 2**).[8] The mortality rate were measured separately via subgroup analysis: HF based on clinical findings versus CI and PCWP via right heart catheter. The increase in mortality among patients with compromised peripheral circulations and pulmonary congestions was observed evenly between two

Table 1 Killip classification			
Class	Clinical Findings	Mortality (%)	Management
I	No congestion	<6	• To check volume status and peripheral perfusion (ie, cool extremities, decreased urine output) • If hypovolemic state, consider volume resuscitation
II	S3, rales	<17	• To check volume status • If hypervolemic state, consider using diuretics
III	Acute pulmonary edema	38	• To check cardiac function and volume status • If systolic function is impaired, consider using inotropes with diuretics • Consider noninvasive positive pulmonary pressure support devices (ie, CPAP or Bi-level PAP)
IV	Cardiogenic shock	81	• Consider both inotropes and diuretics • If hemodynamic improvement is not achieved, consider starting mechanical circulatory support devices (ie, intra-aortic balloon pump, percutaneous cardiopulmonary support, or temporary left ventricular assist device)

Abbreviations: Bi-level PAP, bi-level positive airway pressure; CPAP, continue positive airway pressure; S3, third heart sounds.

Table 2
Clinical findings and Forrester classification

Class	Clinical Findings	Mortality (%)	Hemodynamics	Mortality (%)
I	No evidence of heart failure	1	PCWP $\leq$18 mm Hg CI $\geq$2.2 L/min/m^2	3
II	Pulmonary congestion	11	PCWP >18 mm Hg CI $\geq$2.2 L/min/m^2	9
III	Isolated peripheral hypoperfusion	18	PCWP $\leq$18 mm Hg CI <2.2 L/min/m^2	23
IV	Shock with rales, tissue and end-organ hypoperfusion	60	PCWP >18 mm Hg CI <2.2 L/min/m^2	51

Abbreviations: CI, cardiac index; PCWP, pulmonary capillary wedge pressure.

studies. Thus, both Killip classification and Forrester classification showed increase in mortality with worsening congestion.

Nohria-Stevenson Classification

Another noninvasive classification method was developed by Norhia and Stevenson for HF; they categorized patients by the severity of congestions (ie, orthopnea, hepatojugular reflux, peripheral edema, rales) and the severity of hypoperfusion (the presence of a narrow pulse pressure <25%, cool extremities, pulsus alternans, and so forth) (**Fig. 1**).[9] Their classification also showed a strong correlation with New York Heart Association (NYHA) classification. Patients in group C (Wet-Cold) had the highest mortality rate with a hazard ratio (HR) of 3.66 (*P*<.01) when compared with control group A (Dry-Warm). When these patients were stratified based on NYHA classes, groups B and C were composed largely of NYHA III/IV. Group C patients who were classified in NYHA III/IV had HR of 2.73 (*P*<.009).[9] To categorize patients with HF by

the Norhia-Stevenson classification is a sophisticated approach in the clinical setting as it provides guidance on immediate medical therapy without any invasive measures to assess their hemodynamic status and allows to estimate their prognosis.

Clinical Scenarios

A multidisciplinary team of cardiology, emergency medicine, and critical care medicine developed a tool called Clinical Scenarios to provide recommendation on the initial step of acute HF management.[10] These were meant to be recommendations to augment current guidelines especially during prehospital condition and presentation in the first 6 to 12 hours.[10] There are 5 different types of Clinical Scenarios and each has specific recommendations on immediate medical therapy regimens (**Table 3**).[10,11] In addition to these findings, Clinical Scenarios also emphasizes assessing the renal function and urine output of the patients to evaluate their perfusion status.[10] Early categorization of HF at their prehospitalization

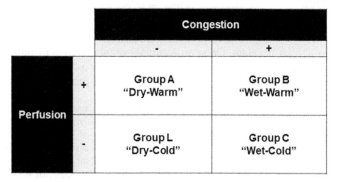

Fig. 1. Nohria-Stevenson classification. The Nohria-Stevenson classification divides heart failure populations based on presence or absence of hypoperfusion and congestion. Group A is Dry-Warm where patients have adequate peripheral circulation and no signs of congestion. Group B is Wet-Warm where patients have adequate circulation as well as signs and symptoms of congestion. Group L is Dry-Cold where patients have poor peripheral circulation but no congestion. Group C is Wet-Cold where there is hypoperfusion and signs and symptoms of congestion.

- **Criteria of Low Perfusion:** cool extremities, *pulsus alternans*, narrow pulse pressure, hypotension, decreased urine output or kidney function.

- **Criteria of Congestion:** paroxysmal nocturnal dyspnea, orthopnea, leg edema, S3, rales, jugular venous pressure,

Table 3
Clinical scenarios

Class	Characteristics	Treatment[a]

CS 1	SBP >140 mm Hg
	  Abrupt onset
	  Predominantly diffuse pulmonary edema
	  Minimal systemic edema, increased filling pressure
	  Preserved LVEF
		Noninvasive ventilation
		Nitrates (ie, nitroglycerine spray)
		+/− Diuretics (use if volume overloaded, but it may be rare)

CS 2	SBP 100–140 mm Hg
	  Gradual onset
	  Predominantly systemic edema
	    Minimum pulmonary edema
	  Chronically increased filling pressure
		Noninvasive ventilation
		Nitrates
		+/− Diuretics

CS 3	SBP <100 mm Hg
	  Rapid or gradual
	  Signs of hypoperfusion
	  Minimal pulmonary or systemic edema
	  Subtypes:
	  I. Hypoperfusion or cardiogenic shock
	  II. No hypoperfusion or cardiogenic shock
		Initial fluid challenge if there is no signs of overt volume overload
		Inotropes (ie, dobutamine, dopamine, milrinone)
		Vasopressors if SBP <90 mm Hg or in cardiogenic shock

CS 4	Acute coronary syndrome
	  Acute symptoms and signs of acute heart failure
	  Evidence of ACS
		Noninvasive ventilation, nitrates, cardiac catheterization
		ASA, heparin, reperfusion therapy

CS 5	Right heart failure
	  Acute or gradual onset without pulmonary edema
	  Signs of RV dysfunction
		Diuretics if SBP >90 mm Hg and signs of volume overload
		Inotropes if SBP <90 mm Hg

Abbreviations: ACS, acute coronary syndrome; ASA, aspirin; CS, clinical scenario; LVEF, left ventricular ejection fraction; RV, right ventricle; SBP, systolic blood pressure.
[a] Treatment is recommended therapy for the initial 90 to 120 min after hospital admissions.

is beneficial to facilitate a targeted treatment that is tailored for their hemodynamic status and pathophysiology from early-stage of diagnosis.

PHYSICAL EXAMINATION WITH POSITIVE AND NEGATIVE LIKELIHOOD RATIOS FOR POSTTEST PROBABILITY

To increase the accuracy and precision of patient assessment derived from physical examinations, understanding likelihood ratio, sensitivity, and specificity of each of the key examination findings is a powerful insight. The likelihood ratio is used to estimate how likely a patient may have a disease with a given pretest probability. Sensitivity and specificity are equally helpful in either ruling in or out diagnoses (**Fig. 2**).[12] The positive likelihood ratio is used for positive test results, whereas the negative likelihood ratio is applied for negative test results. Once an examiner obtains values of pretest probability and likelihood ratio for a distinct physical examination finding, the posttest probability can be

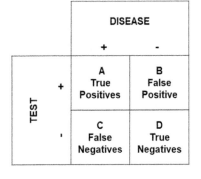
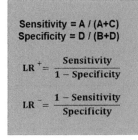

$$\text{Sensitivity} = A / (A+C)$$
$$\text{Specificity} = D / (B+D)$$

$$LR^{+} = \frac{\text{Sensitivity}}{1 - \text{Specificity}}$$

$$LR^{-} = \frac{1 - \text{Sensitivity}}{\text{Specificity}}$$

Fig. 2. Sensitivity, specificity, and likelihood ratio. Sensitivity is used to test for a probability of having positive test if one has a disease. Specificity is to test a probability of resulting in negative test if one does not have a disease. Likelihood ratio (LR) is classified by positive LR or negative LR. The positive LR shows by how much having a positive test will increase the probability of truly having a disease.

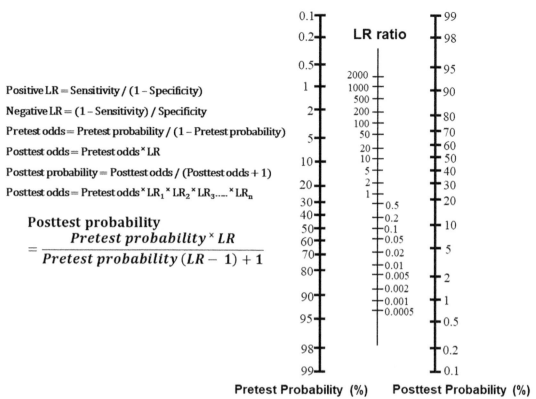

Positive LR = Sensitivity / (1 – Specificity)

Negative LR = (1 – Sensitivity) / Specificity

Pretest odds = Pretest probability / (1 – Pretest probability)

Posttest odds = Pretest odds × LR

Posttest probability = Posttest odds / (Posttest odds + 1)

Posttest odds = Pretest odds × LR_1 × LR_2 × LR_3 .... × LR_n

$$\text{Posttest probability} = \frac{Pretest\ probability \times LR}{Pretest\ probability\ (LR - 1) + 1}$$

Pretest Probability (%)   Posttest Probability (%)

Fig. 3. Posttest probability estimation with likelihood ratio (LR). The multiplicative relationship between pretest probability and likelihood ratio can provide an estimated posttest probability, which can be extrapolated from a linear line drawn between the 2 values of pretest probability and LR in a monogram (*right*).

extrapolated based on their multiplicative relationships (**Fig. 3**). The posttest probabilities can be obtained by the following steps:

Positive Likelihood ratio = Sensitivity/(1 – Specificity)   (1)

Negative Likelihood ratio = (1 – Sensitivity)/Specificity   (2)

Pretest odds = Pretest probability/(1 – Pretest probability)   (3)

Posttest odds = Pretest odds × Likelihood ratio   (4)

Posttest probability = Posttest odds/(Posttest odds + 1)   (5)

Through step (1)–(5), the posttest probability can be calculated (6):

Posttest probability =

$$\frac{Pretest\ probability \times Likelihood\ ratio}{Pretest\ probability\ (Likelihood\ ratio - 1) + 1}$$ (6)

In a clinical setting, a monogram is accessibly available to calculate the posttest probability (see **Fig. 3**). The posttest probability with a higher precision is also deducible by multiplying pretest probability and several likelihood ratios (LR). This relationship of coupling with a sequence of events is known as a Markov process or Markov chains (7).[13,14]

Posttest odds = Pretest odds × LR_1 × LR_2 × LR_3..... × LR_n (7)

The LR of distinct physical findings correlated with presented illness, such as wheeze, S3, or hepatojugular reflex seen in HF can be summated to provide more definite posttest probability. The LR for commonly seen physical findings from HF are summarized in **Table 4**.[15]

VITAL SIGNS AND HEMODYNAMICS
Heart Rate, Blood Pressure, and Proportional Pulse Pressure

The evaluation of vital signs in patients with acute HF is a crucial step to identify the severity of decompensation. The incidence of tachyarrhythmia and brady-arrhythmia will likely increase if heart rate >120/min or less than 60/min.[16]

Table 4
Likelihood ratio of key findings in patients with heart failure

		Sensitivity	Specificity	LR$^+$ (95% CI)	LR$^-$ (95% CI)
History	Heart failure	60	90	5.8 (4.1–8.0)	0.45 (0.38–0.53)
	Myocardial infarction	40	87	3.1 (2.0–4.9)	0.69 (0.58–0.82)
	Coronary artery disease	52	70	1.8 (1.1–2.8)	0.68 (0.48–0.96)
	Dyslipidemia	23	87	1.7 (0.43–6.9)	0.89(0.69–1.1)
	Diabetes mellitus	28	83	1.7 (1.0–2.7)	0.86 (0.73–1.0)
	Hypertension	60	56	1.4 (1.1–1.7)	0.71(0.55–0.93)
Symptoms	Paroxysmal nocturnal dyspnea	41	84	2.6 (1.5–4.5)	0.70 (0.54–0.91)
	Orthopnea	50	77	2.2 (1.2–3.9)	0.65 (0.45–0.92)
	Edema	51	76	2.1 (0.92–5.0)	0.64 (0.39–1.1)
	Dyspnea on exertion	84	34	1.3 (1.2–1.4)	0.48 (0.35–0.67)
	Fatigue/weight gain	31	70	1.0 (0.74–1.4)	0.99 (0.85–1.1)
Physical examination	Heart S3 (ventricular filling gallop)	13	99	11 (4.9–25.0)	0.88 (0.83–0.94)
	Abdominojugular reflux	24	96	6.4 (0.81–51.0)	0.79 (0.62–1.0)
	Jugular venous distension	39	92	5.1 (3.2–7.9)	0.66 (0.57–0.77)
	Rales	60	78	2.8 (1.9–4.1)	0.51 (0.37–0.70)
	Any heart murmurs	27	90	2.6 (1.7–4.1)	0.81 (0.73–0.90)
	Lower extremity edema	50	78	2.3 (1.5–3.7)	0.64 (0.47–0.87)
	Valsalva maneuver	73	65	2.1 (1.0–4.2)	0.41 (0.17–1.0)
	SBP < 100 mm Hg	6	97	2.0 (0.60–6.6)	0.97 (0.91–1.0)
	Heart S4 (atrial gallop)	5	97	1.6 (0.47–5.5)	0.98 (0.93–1.0)
	SBP ≥ 150 mm Hg	28	73	1.0 (0.69–1.6)	0.99 (0.84–1.2)

Abbreviations: CI, confidence interval; LR$^+$, positive likelihood ratio; LR$^-$, negative likelihood ratio; SBP, systolic blood pressure.

Adapted from Wang CS, FitzGerald JM, Schulzer M, et al. Does this dyspneic patient in the emergency department have congestive heart failure? JAMA 2005;294(15):1950; with permission.

Ideally, blood pressure (BP) needs to be measured in a seated position with the patient's arm at the level of the heart to obtain accurate measurements. Appropriate cuff size also needs to be used since a smaller cuff can overestimate the BP. Orthostatic hypotension, which is defined by decrease in systolic BP greater than 20 mm Hg or diastolic BP greater than 10 mm Hg from supine to standing position, indicates hypoperfusion or autonomic insufficiency.[17] Cardiogenic shock is diagnosed when systolic BP is less than 90 mm Hg.[18] Proportional pulse pressure derived from (systolic BP – diastolic BP)/systolic BP is used to assess cardiac function in association with CI. If proportional pulse pressure is less than 25%, the CI will be less than 2.2 L/min/m^2; whereas, when proportional pulse pressure is greater than 25%, CI will be greater than 2.2 L/min/m^2.[19] This relationship between proportional pulse pressure and CI was shown to have sensitivity of 91% and specificity of 83%.[18] Hypoperfusion evident by low proportional pulse pressure is caused by reduced systemic perfusion from decreased cardiac output; this is equivalent to a hemodynamic profile seen in the Wet-Cold group from the Nohria-Stevenson classification, which showed higher mortality than other groups. Hence, when reduction in proportional pulse pressure is observed, an immediate response with inotrope to increase contractility and nitrates for lessening afterload is necessary to improve cardiac output and systemic circulation.

Respiratory Rate, Bendopnea, and Trepopnea

Patients may exhibit tachypnea with respiratory rate greater than 18 breaths per minute derived by hypoxemia or pulmonary edema. Severe hypoxemia is defined as SpO2 less than 90% or partial arterial oxygen pressure (PaO2) less than 60 mm Hg, which generally requires prompt respiratory support either with noninvasive or invasive methods.[16] In addition to orthopnea or paroxysmal nocturnal dyspnea, bendopnea, which is dyspnea worsened by bending forward, or trepopnea, which is dyspnea noted in the lateral decubitus position, may be reported by patients.

Bendopnea is caused by higher PCWP and left ventricular (LV) filling pressure surpassing the threshold to trigger symptoms of dyspnea. It is also independent of obesity or a large waist circumference.[20] In a bending position, the filling pressure increases secondary from high intrathoracic pressure. There is only a small reduction in CI from supine to bending position, thus a difference in CI is shown to be noncontributary to bendopnea.[20]

Trepopnea is observed especially when patients are lying in the left lateral decubitus position.[21] One of many theories that have been proposed is that it is due to decreased diastolic function from externally compressed LV by lying on the left side causing symptoms of dyspnea.[21] However, a clear mechanism of trepopnea is still not known.

Cardiopulmonary Examination

In general, patients with acute HF will exhibit signs of congestion, including increased jugular venous pressure (JVP), peripheral edema commonly noted in bilateral lower extremities, presence of rales or crackles on lung examinations, displaced point of maximum impulse especially if there is a concomitant cardiomegaly, and the presence of a third heart sound (S3) (**Fig. 4**G). S3 is heard best at the apex using the bell of a stethoscope. S3 is heard during early diastole and it indicates rapid filling into the left ventricle. Although its sensitivity (32%–73%) and specificity (42%–99%) tend to vary across different studies, S3 is a good predictor of increased left ventricular end diastolic pressure (LVEDP) greater than 15 mm Hg and reduced systolic ventricular function.[15] The probability of HF seen with the presence of S3 was reported with an LR of 11 (95% CI, 4.9–25.0) in 22 studies evaluated in emergency department settings.[15] It is also associated with increased mortality and worse prognosis when concomitant cardiovascular diseases, such as myocardial infarction, are present.[15] Moreover, S3 itself is a poor indicator of ejection fraction as it reflects diastolic function and not systolic function, hence it is not used to assess for innate cardiac function. Although detection of S3 can be variable due to differences in individual skills, the presence of S3 could indicate worse mortality and LV function, subsequently requiring careful management and close monitoring. The fourth heart sound (S4) is low frequency sound at the end of diastole and is caused by vibration of the LV during atrial contraction (**Fig. 4**H). S4 is associated with low LV compliance.

Percussion of the heart border is helpful not only to detect cardiomegaly but also to assess LVEDV. Normally, the changes from resonant to dullness on percussion can be appreciated about 6 cm lateral to the left sternum border. If the sound of dullness is detected over 10.5 cm in the left fifth intercostal space, it can indicate increased LVEDV

with a sensitivity of 91.3% and a specificity of 30.3%.[22] If a patient's apical impulse is greater than 3 cm found in the lateral decubitus position, it can indicate increased LVEDV or the presence of an LV mass with a sensitivity of 100% and a specificity of 40%.[22]

Jugular Venous Pressure

The internal jugular vein (IJV) is a better estimation of central venous pressure as it is directly above right atrium (RA) and nonvalved vein as opposed to the external jugular vein (EJV). However, the EJV is much more accessible in clinical practice, hence it can be used as an aid for volume status assessment. Increased JVP has shown a correlation with increased LVEDP noted on previous right heart catheterization studies.[23] In fact, the presence of JVP was reported to have PCWP $\geq$ 18 mm Hg with a sensitivity of 81% and a specificity of 80%.[24] To perform JVP examination, a patient should be examined at the head of a bed angled at 30° to 45° with his or her neck turned, relaxing the sternocleidomastoid muscle to improve visualization. It is also important to differentiate from the carotid artery; the jugular vein is nonpalpable and has 2 cycles of crests.[25] Using a pen light for better visualization or a sticky note to monitor for oscillation to demonstrate an IJV waveform may be helpful for identification. To estimate JVP, the distance from the intersection between sternal angle to visible pulsation of IJV is measured. An additional 5 cm H_2O is added to account for the pressure estimated for RA. If this is greater than 7 to 8 cm, it indicates increased central venous pressure.[25] If JVP is not visible, performing hepatojugular reflux by pressing the abdomen to increase venous return may cause increase in venous pressure.

Other Findings

The European Society of Cardiology guidelines from 2016 stated that increased JVP, hepatojugular reflux, S3, and laterally displaced apical impulse were specific signs and symptoms of HF.[26] However, in patients with coexisting comorbidities of chronic lung disease, kidney disease, or obesity, precise assessment of volume status may become more challenging.[26] In fact, most patients in clinical practice will have multiple comorbidities. Hence, acknowledging additional key physical examination findings may be helpful to support the diagnosis of HF. For instance, central cyanosis indicates significant right to left shunt in cardiopulmonary circulation and it is often accompanied with distal limb clubbing. On the other hand, peripheral cyanosis is more indicative of severe

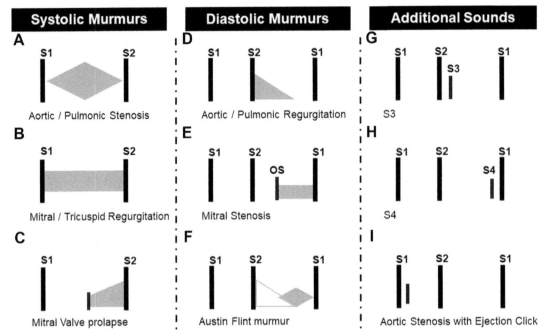

Fig. 4. Systolic and diastolic heart murmur. (*A*) Aortic/pulmonic stenosis: systolic ejection murmur, crescendo-decrescendo heard best at the right upper sternal border. (*B*) Mitral/tricuspid regurgitation: mitral regurgitation is a high-pitched, low intensity, holosystolic heard best at the apex. Tricuspid regurgitation is low intensity, low pitch and heard best at the left lower sternal border. (*C*) Mitral valve prolapse: holosystolic murmur with none-jection click heard at the apex. (*D*) Aortic/pulmonic regurgitation: a soft early diastolic murmur is heard in acute regurgitation at the left sternal border. In chronic aortic regurgitation, a louder decrescendo diastolic murmur can be appreciated. Pulmonic regurgitation will be soft, decrescendo, diastolic murmur heard best at the left second or third intercostal spaces. (*E*) Mitral stenosis: the sound of an opening snap (OS) is followed by a high-pitched blowing decrescendo diastolic murmur best appreciated at the apex. (*F*) Austin Flint murmur: this has a soft, low frequency sound that diminishes with decreasing jet flow volume during diastole. (*G*) S3: additional heart sound is heard soon after S2. (*H*) S4: additional heart sound is heard at presystole or before S1. (*I*) Aortic stenosis with ejection click: a high-pitched sound followed soon after S1, indicating a rapid blood flow during opening of stenotic valve.

vasoconstrictions resulted from marked hypoperfusion with heart failure. Ascites can be present with acute HF but is nonspecific as it can be present with nephrotic syndromes or cirrhosis. Anasarca can also be seen if there is coexisting hypoalbuminemia but otherwise it is seldomly noted. If a patient has concomitant chronic obstructive pulmonary disease, pulmonary hypertension, or kyphoscoliosis, this can lead to right heart failure with signs of congestion. Right upper quadrant pain can be caused by congestive hepatopathy. These findings are not specific for HF but are valuable in supporting the diagnosis acute HF.

VALVULAR DYSFUNCTION-RELATED HEART FAILURE

Valvular defects can also affect the prognosis of acute HF. It is important to consider the chronicity of the valvular defect as it can remain stable without decompensation or cause acute HF, especially in relation to acute ischemic injury.[27] In cardiac

auscultation, there may be variability in detecting cardiac murmurs due to differences in patients body habitus, pulses, and examiners' skills. Cardiac murmurs often signify the presence of valvular diseases and they may play a role in the causes of acute HF, requiring specific therapies. Cardiac murmurs can be classified as either systolic, diastolic, or continuous murmur. The nearest points of auscultation where the murmurs were heard the loudest imply a defect in that specific valve associated with the location of the pericardium. Valvular defects can be stenosis, regurgitation, or others (**Fig. 4**G-I).

Aortic Stenosis

The most common cause of aortic stenosis (AS) is calcification of leaflets causing restricted movements of valves.[28] Age-related stenosis can manifest as a sequala of aortic sclerosis. Other causes include a bicuspid valve, which is often seen in the fifth or sixth decades; this is because of poor susceptibility to degenerative changes and some genetic components.[29] About 30% of population born with bicuspid valve will develop aortic stenosis. In addition to symptoms of angina or syncope, AS can manifest as congestive HF.[30] Auscultation reveals systolic ejection murmur radiating to the carotid artery. Murmur is described as a crescendo-decrescendo sound with late-peaking at mid systole, which is heard best at the right upper sternal border (**Fig. 4**A). An examiner may hear an ejection click, a high-pitched sound followed soon after S1, indicating a rapid blood flow during opening of the stenotic valve; this is more commonly observed in bicuspid valve-related stenosis (**Fig. 4**I). The peak of ejection murmur will be further delayed if the stenosis is severe. On the contrary, the loudness of the murmur does not indicate the severity of stenosis. Carotid artery examination may show parvus tardus, which is slow and delayed carotid upstroke secondary to prolonged ejection from limited outflow through aortic valves.[30] In severe AS, the second heart sound will be delayed and soft; if only the sound of P2 is heard, the aortic valve maybe too restricted to close rapidly.[30]

Aortic Regurgitation

The main cause of aortic regurgitation can be divided into 2 types; root dilation or leaflet pathology. For example, aortic semilunar valves can become dysfunctional in the setting of infective endocarditis, bicuspid valves, or collagen vascular disease, eg, lupus and prolapse. On the other hand, aortic root dilatation can be associated with Marfan syndrome, hypertension, aortic dissection, syphilis-related aortitis, and others. Auscultation of aortic regurgitation defers between acute findings or chronic findings; a soft early diastolic murmur is heard in acute regurgitation, whereas a louder decrescendo diastolic murmur can be appreciated in the chronic setting.[31] Soft S1 may indicate mitral valve preclosure or a new atrioventricular block, which is often considered to be a life-threatening event when found concomitantly with aortic regurgitation. These murmurs can be intensified when the patient is sitting upward and leaning forward (**Fig. 4**D). With root enlargement or other secondary types of aortic regurgitation, the murmur will show radiation down to left lower sternal border.[32] The sensitivity and specificity of auscultation of diastolic murmur identifying the presence of aortic regurgitation were 73% and 92%, respectively.[33] The Austin Flint murmur is a diastolic murmur that can be appreciated at the apex with the bell of the stethoscope lightly held against the skin (**Fig. 4**F).

Similarly to other murmurs, the intensity can vary with physical maneuvers, that is hand grip or squatting.[34] This murmur is caused by jet flow from aortic regurgitation that is abutting to a closing mitral valve heard as rambling of diastolic murmur. It can be mistaken for mitral stenosis (MS) but they are differentiable by carefully listening to the intensity and duration of the murmur; Austin Flint murmur has a soft, low frequency sound that diminishes with decreasing jet flow volume.[35,36] There are other cardinal physical examination findings, seen in carotid artery with aortic regurgitation: Corrigan pulse, a sharp rise followed by a rapid decline in carotid pulse, and pulsus bisferiens, first strong upward pulse and second gradual downward stroke. In addition, Quinke's pulse, nail bed appearing plethoric in systole and blanching in diastole, or head-bobbing known as de Musset's sign may be also appreciated.[32]

Mitral Stenosis

The incidence of MS has significantly declined with reduced incidence of rheumatic heart disease. However, MS still remains the most common cause of rheumatic heart disease, and MS due to degenerative changes is relatively rare.[37] A pause heard soon after S2 corresponds to the isovolumetric relaxation phase. The sound of an opening snap (OS) is followed by a high-pitched blowing decrescendo diastolic murmur that can be appreciated at the apex (**Fig. 4**E). It is best heard at the lateral decubitus position to bring the heart closer to the chest wall and by using the bell of the stethoscope. The sooner the sound of OS is heard after S2, the more severe the stenosis is. This is because of increased pressure in left atrium (LA) allowing the mitral valves to snap open much faster. In fact, atrial fibrillation is commonly found in patients with MS due to an increased LA pressure causing LA dilatation. In atrial fibrillation, the diastolic rumble, also known as presystolic murmur, is usually louder and starts later than in patients in sinus rhythm. This is because the atrial contraction at the end of diastole increases flow against the closing mitral valve, which subsequently amplify the sound of the murmur.[38] With increased LA pressure, a loud P2 sound, which signifies closure of the pulmonic valve, may be found in these patients. If patients develop pulmonary hypertension, right ventricular heave, or mitral facies, cutaneous venous dilation causing red/purple of the face can be seen. Concomitant presence of pulmonary valve insufficiency secondary to MS-induced pulmonary hypertension may cause diastolic murmur at the left upper sternal border

(LUSB) known as Graham Steell murmur. However, this can be mistaken with aortic regurgitation and may be less prevalent than the previously reported incidence, 10% to 15% of the population with severe MS.[39] If other clinical findings, such as Corrigan pulse or pulsus bisferiens is present, diastolic murmur at the LUSB is more likely to suggest the presence of aortic regurgitation. On the other hand, if the patient has signs of pulmonary hypertension, such as right sternal heave, loud S2 sound, or right ventricular hypertrophy noted in EKG or echocardiogram, diastolic murmur can indicate Graham Steell murmur.[40]

Mitral Regurgitation

The cause of mitral regurgitation can vary similarly to MS. In the acute setting, ischemic mitral regurgitation caused by myocardial infarction induced papillary muscle rupture and/or displacement, rupture of mitral chordae tendineae secondary to underlying connective tissue disease, such as mitral valve prolapse syndrome, Marfan syndrome, or as sequalae of chronic rheumatic disease or infective endocarditis can occur.[31,41]

In patients with mitral regurgitation, patients normally present with a high-pitched, low intensity, holosystolic murmur heard best at the apex (see Fig. 4B).[42] It increases in intensity with maneuvers of hand grip with sensitivity of 68% and specificity of 92%. Historically speaking, the intensity of murmur was found to diminish by inhalation of amyl nitrite (80% sensitivity and 90% specificity).[43] In the case of papillary muscle or chordae tendinea rupture, the patient may have a harsh holosystolic decrescendo murmur best heard at the apex radiating to the axilla.[42] Nonejection click can also be heard in the presence of mitral valve prolapse (Fig. 4C). The click will be heard closer to S1 in a standing position due to decreased preload and increase afterload, whereas it will be heard later in systole in a squatting position. If S3 is heard with diastolic murmur from mitral regurgitation, it likely suggests greater mean LV volume secondary to restricted filling and severe regurgitation. Primary LV dysfunction was also reported is patients with mitral regurgitation and presence of S3.[44]

Tricuspid Regurgitation

Most tricuspid regurgitation is due to secondary causes, such as enlarged right ventricle (RV) or RA, causing dilatation of the tricuspid annulus and displacement of papillary muscles. Increase in pulmonary pressure from severe pulmonary hypertension, and RV dysfunction with or without left heart disease can lead to dilatation of RV, subsequently causing regurgitation through the tricuspid valves. In fact, most adults will develop a small degree of tricuspid regurgitation with aging.[45] Along with systolic murmur, parasternal heave, distinct jugular pulse, hepatomegaly, and peripheral edema maybe present, but often tricuspid regurgitation is difficult to detect on physical examination. Murmur of tricuspid regurgitation is often of low intensity, low pitch, and heard best at the left lower sternal border (see Fig. 4B).[46,47] The specificity and sensitivity of tricuspid murmur are 100% and 66%, respectively, if found simultaneously with hepatojugular reflux.[48]

CARDIAC TAMPONADE

Cardiac tamponade requires immediate attention to correct hemodynamic disturbances from decreased cardiac output and ventricular filling by increased intrapericardial pressure impeding sufficient ventricular filling. Cardiac tamponade occurs when pericardial fluid accumulates and exceeds a pressure greater than that of central venous pressure.[49] The Beck triad is a collection of physical findings: (1) muffled heart sounds, (2) increased JVP, and (3) hypotension. The increase in central venous pressure should be equivalent to the pressure in the intrapericardium because of fluid accumulation.[50] Other associated findings include dyspnea (sensitivity of 87%–89%), tachycardia (sensitivity of 77%), pulsus paradoxus (sensitivity of 82%), increased JVP (sensitivity of 76%).[49] Pulsus paradoxus showed a positive LR of 5.9 with a systolic BP difference of 12 mm Hg, but a positive LR of 3.3 with a systolic BP difference of 10 mm Hg. When a difference of 10 mm Hg was observed, cardiac tamponade was considered to be less likely given its negative LR of 0.03.[49] If these features are found and suspicion for cardiac tamponade is high, an emergent echocardiogram followed by pericardiocentesis may be warranted.

PHYSICAL EXAMINATION AND RIGHT HEART CATHETERIZATION

Right heart catheterization is the only absolute measure to obtain true values of hemodynamics in HF patients. However, catheterization is invasive and not feasible to perform in every patient who presents to hospital for HF symptoms. The ESCAPE trial showed that there was no difference in mortality among patients who received medical therapies after undergoing pulmonary artery catheter study or patients who received pharmacologic therapy after undergoing clinical assessments only.[51] Stevenson and Perloff[18] showed increased association between increased PCWP ($\geq$22 mm Hg) and cardinal physical examination findings of

HF, such as JVP, leg edema, rales, and reduced pulse pressure. Based on these findings, right heart catheterization is useful when hemodynamic measurements are required for critical condition or pharmacotherapy that requires close monitoring. However, right heart catheterization is not required to initiate initial treatment of acute HF as clinical assessment can suffice to provide information on patients' hemodynamic status.

JUGULAR VENOUS WAVEFORMS

The venous waveforms can be measured with catheterization, which provides accurate readings of central venous pressure. The venous pressure can be estimated by measuring the highest pulsation point in IJV from the sternal inflection point, the angle of Louis. However, this is often challenging because of variance in body habitus and positioning.[25] The venous

waveforms during diastole comprises of the *v* wave, which signifies passive atrial filling during diastasis, followed by a *y* descending wave indicating decline in atrial pressure after closure of the tricuspid valve. Next, an *a* wave, which indicates presystolic atrial contraction, is seen. An *x* wave appears immediately after the *a* wave, indicating a fall in atrial pressure along with tricuspid valves suctioned into RV in the first phase of systole. This event is followed by the appearance of waveform *c*, which indicates a mild increase in central venous pressure from the ventricular systole against the closed tricuspid valve (**Fig. 5A**). Abnormal waveform patterns can be helpful to discern changes in filling pressure of RA or RV, providing key information on underlying hemodynamics in patients. For example, the presence of a prominent *a* wave suggests reduced compliance of RV resulting in higher filling pressure. A large *a* wave, known as a cannon *a* wave, occurs

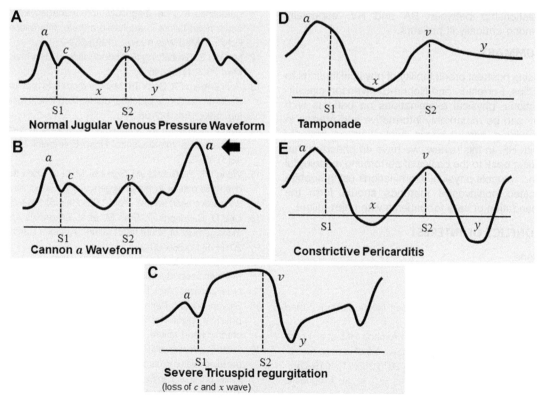

Fig. 5. Jugular venous pressure waveform. (*A*) Normal jugular venous pressure waveform: *a* wave shows presystolic atrial contraction. A *c* wave signifies ventricular systole against closed tricuspid valve. An *x* wave shows a fall in atrial pressure in the first phase of systole. A *v* wave signifies passive atrial filling during diastasis, followed by a *y* descending wave indicating a decline in atrial pressure after closure of the tricuspid valve. (*B*) Cannon *a* waveform: a large *a* wave occurs when the atria contract against a closed tricuspid valve. (*C*) Severe tricuspid regurgitation: a *v* wave merged together with a *c* wave appears with a steep *y* waveform, signifying equalization of filling pressure from retrograde ventricular flow. (*D*) Tamponade: a prominent *x* descent followed by a slow *y* descent are seen in tamponade due to reduction in right atrium pressure during systole and increased right atrium pressure during diastole. (*E*) Constrictive pericarditis: a preserved *x* descent and prominent *y* descent, which can depict W shape morphology, can be seen.

when atria contract against a closed tricuspid valve (**Fig. 5**B). This often indicates the presence of atrioventricular dissociation.[25] In severe tricuspid regurgitation, the *y* waveform will appear steeper, and the *v* wave will be merged together with the *c* wave; this is because of rapid equalization of filling pressure due to retrograde flow from RV into RA (**Fig. 5**C). In cardiac tamponade, a prominent *x* descent and slow *y* descent can be seen, indicating reduction in RA pressure during systole but persistently increased RA pressure during diastole (**Fig. 5**D).[52] The Kussmal sign, a paradoxic increase in JVP during inspiration, may be present if an increased filling pressure is noted in right side chambers because of increased intrapericardial pressure.[52] In constrictive pericarditis, the JVP waveform will show a preserved *x* descent and prominent *y* descent, which can depict W shape morphology (**Fig. 5**E).[52] Thus, central venous pressure evaluation by JVP is useful to precisely estimate the relationship between RA and RV, especially among critically ill patients.

SUMMARY

Using posttest predictability of physical findings to Killips, Forrester, and Nohria-Steavenson classifications, physical examinations on patients with HF can be remarkably informative and precise in providing hemodynamic evaluation on patients with HF. In this review, we have emphasized that going back to the basics of performing meaningful and valuable physical examinations using sophisticated noninvasive methods should form the foundation of care for patients with heart failure.

CONFLICT OF INTEREST

None.

REFERENCES

1. Jessup M, Brozena S. Heart failure. N Engl J Med 2003;348(20):2007–18.
2. Chan PS, Nallamothu BK, Krumholz HM, et al. Long-term outcomes in elderly survivors of in-hospital cardiac arrest. N Engl J Med 2013;368(11):1019–26.
3. Khot UN, Jia G, Moliterno DJ, et al. Prognostic importance of physical examination for heart failure in non-ST-elevation acute coronary syndromes: the enduring value of Killip classification. JAMA 2003; 290(16):2174–81.
4. Stevenson WG, Stevenson LW, Middlekauff HR, et al. Improving survival for patients with advanced heart failure: a study of 737 consecutive patients. J Am Coll Cardiol 1995;26(6):1417–23.
5. El-Menyar A, Zubaid M, AlMahmeed W, et al. Killip classification in patients with acute coronary syndrome: insight from a multicenter registry. Am J Emerg Med 2012;30(1):97–103.
6. McKee PA, Castelli WP, McNamara PM, et al. The natural history of congestive heart failure: the Framingham study. N Engl J Med 1971;285(26):1441–6.
7. Killip T 3rd, Kimball JT. Treatment of myocardial infarction in a coronary care unit. A two year experience with 250 patients. Am J Cardiol 1967;20(4):457–64.
8. Forrester JS, Diamond GA, Swan HJ. Correlative classification of clinical and hemodynamic function after acute myocardial infarction. Am J Cardiol 1977;39(2):137–45.
9. Nohria A, Tsang SW, Fang JC, et al. Clinical assessment identifies hemodynamic profiles that predict outcomes in patients admitted with heart failure. J Am Coll Cardiol 2003;41(10):1797–804.
10. Mebazaa A, Gheorghiade M, Pina IL, et al. Practical recommendations for prehospital and early in-hospital management of patients presenting with acute heart failure syndromes. Crit Care Med 2008;36(1 Suppl):S129–39.
11. Mebazaa A. Current ESC/ESICM and ACCF/AHA guidelines for the diagnosis and management of acute heart failure in adults—are there differences? Pol Arch Med Wewn 2009;119(9):569–73.
12. McGee S. Simplifying likelihood ratios. J Gen Intern Med 2002;17(8):646–9.
13. Sonnenberg FA, Beck JR. Markov models in medical decision making: a practical guide. Med Decis Making 1993;13(4):322–38.
14. Tom E, Schulman KA. Mathematical models in decision analysis. Infect Control Hosp Epidemiol 1997; 18(1):65–73.
15. Wang CS, FitzGerald JM, Schulzer M, et al. Does this dyspneic patient in the emergency department have congestive heart failure? JAMA 2005;294(15):1944–56.
16. Ural D, Cavusoglu Y, Eren M, et al. Diagnosis and management of acute heart failure. Anatol J Cardiol 2015;15(11):860–89.
17. Luukinen H, Koski K, Laippala P, et al. Prognosis of diastolic and systolic orthostatic hypotension in older persons. Arch Intern Med 1999;159(3):273–80.
18. Stevenson LW, Perloff JK. The limited reliability of physical signs for estimating hemodynamics in chronic heart failure. JAMA 1989;261(6):884–8.
19. Petrie CJ, Ponikowski P, Metra M, et al. Proportional pulse pressure relates to cardiac index in stabilized acute heart failure patients. Clin Exp Hypertens 2018;40(7):637–43.
20. Thibodeau JT, Turer AT, Gualano SK, et al. Characterization of a novel symptom of advanced heart failure: bendopnea. JACC Heart Fail 2014;2(1):24–31.
21. de Araujo BS, Reichert R, Eifer DA, et al. Trepopnea may explain right-sided pleural effusion in patients with decompensated heart failure. Am J Emerg Med 2012;30(6):925–31.e2.
22. Heckerling PS, Wiener SL, Wolfkiel CJ, et al. Accuracy and reproducibility of precordial percussion and palpation for detecting increased left

ventricular end-diastolic volume and mass. A comparison of physical findings and ultrafast computed tomography of the heart. JAMA 1993; 270(16):1943–8.

23. Drazner MH, Rame JE, Stevenson LW, et al. Prognostic importance of elevated jugular venous pressure and a third heart sound in patients with heart failure. N Engl J Med 2001;345(8):574–81.

24. Butman SM, Ewy GA, Standen JR, et al. Bedside cardiovascular examination in patients with severe chronic heart failure: importance of rest or inducible jugular venous distension. J Am Coll Cardiol 1993; 22(4):968–74.

25. Chua Chiaco JM, Parikh NI, Fergusson DJ. The jugular venous pressure revisited. Cleve Clin J Med 2013;80(10):638–44.

26. Ponikowski P, Voors AA, Anker SD, et al. 2016 ESC guidelines for the diagnosis and treatment of acute and chronic heart failure: the task force for the diagnosis and treatment of acute and chronic heart failure of the European Society of Cardiology (ESC) developed with the special contribution of the Heart Failure Association (HFA) of the ESC. Eur Heart J 2016;37(27):2129–200.

27. Maisel AS, Gilpin EA, Klein L, et al. The murmur of papillary muscle dysfunction in acute myocardial infarction: clinical features and prognostic implications. Am Heart J 1986;112(4):705–11.

28. Cary T, Pearce J. Aortic stenosis: pathophysiology, diagnosis, and medical management of nonsurgical patients. Crit Care Nurse 2013;33(2):58–72.

29. Lindman BR, Clavel MA, Mathieu P, et al. Calcific aortic stenosis. Nat Rev Dis Primers 2016;2:16006.

30. Aronow WS. Valvular aortic stenosis in the elderly. Cardiol Rev 2007;15(5):217–25.

31. Mokadam NA, Stout KK, Verrier ED. Management of acute regurgitation in left-sided cardiac valves. Tex Heart Inst J 2011;38(1):9–19.

32. Harvey WP. Cardiac pearls. Dis Mon 1994;40(2):41–113.

33. Grayburn PA, Smith MD, Handshoe R, et al. Detection of aortic insufficiency by standard echocardiography, pulsed Doppler echocardiography, and auscultation. A comparison of accuracies. Ann Intern Med 1986;104(5):599–605.

34. Sternbach G, Varon J. Austin Flint: on cardiac murmurs. J Emerg Med 1993;11(3):313–5.

35. Reddy PS, Curtiss EI, Salerni R, et al. Sound pressure correlates of the Austin Flint murmur. An intracardiac sound study. Circulation 1976;53(2):210–7.

36. Schocken DD, Arrieta MI, Leaverton PE, et al. Prevalence and mortality rate of congestive heart failure in the United States. J Am Coll Cardiol 1992;20(2): 301–6.

37. Horstkotte D, Niehues R, Strauer BE. Pathomorphological aspects, aetiology and natural history of acquired mitral valve stenosis. Eur Heart J 1991; 12(Suppl B):55–60.

38. Toutouzas P, Koidakis A, Velimezis A, et al. Mechanism of diastolic rumble and presystolic murmur in mitral stenosis. Br Heart J 1974;36(11):1096–105.

39. Runco V, Levin HS, Vahabzadeh H, et al. Basal diastolic murmurs in rheumatic heart disease: intracardiac phonocardiography and cineangiography. Am Heart J 1968;75(2):153–61.

40. Cohn KE, Hultgren HN. The Graham-Steell murmur re-evaluated. N Engl J Med 1966;274(9):486–9.

41. Grenadier E, Alpan G, Keidar S, et al. The prevalence of ruptured chordae tendineae in the mitral valve prolapse syndrome. Am Heart J 1983;105(4):603–10.

42. Compostella L, Compostella C, Russo N, et al. Cardiac auscultation for noncardiologists: application in cardiac rehabilitation programs: part I: patients after acute coronary syndromes and heart failure. J Cardiopulm Rehabil Prev 2017;37(5): 315–21.

43. Lembo NJ, Dell'Italia LJ, Crawford MH, et al. Bedside diagnosis of systolic murmurs. N Engl J Med 1988;318(24):1572–8.

44. Tribouilloy CM, Enriquez-Sarano M, Mohty D, et al. Pathophysiologic determinants of third heart sounds: a prospective clinical and Doppler echocardiographic study. Am J Med 2001;111(2):96–102.

45. Zoghbi WA, Adams D, Bonow RO, et al. Recommendations for noninvasive evaluation of native valvular regurgitation: a report from the American Society of Echocardiography developed in collaboration with the Society for Cardiovascular Magnetic Resonance. J Am Soc Echocardiogr 2017;30(4):303–71.

46. Kelley JR, Guntheroth WG. Pansystolic murmur in the newborn: tricuspid regurgitation versus ventricular septal defect. Arch Dis Child 1988;63(10 Spec No):1172–4.

47. Mikami T, Kudo T, Sakurai N, et al. Mechanisms for development of functional tricuspid regurgitation determined by pulsed Doppler and two-dimensional echocardiography. Am J Cardiol 1984; 53(1):160–3.

48. Maisel AS, Atwood JE, Goldberger AL. Hepatojugular reflux: useful in the bedside diagnosis of tricuspid regurgitation. Ann Intern Med 1984; 101(6):781–2.

49. Roy CL, Minor MA, Brookhart MA, et al. Does this patient with a pericardial effusion have cardiac tamponade? JAMA 2007;297(16):1810–8.

50. Beck C. Two cardiac compression triads. JAMA 1935;104(9):714–6.

51. Drazner MH, Hellkamp AS, Leier CV, et al. Value of clinician assessment of hemodynamics in advanced heart failure: the ESCAPE trial. Circ Heart Fail 2008; 1(3):170–7.

52. Asher CR, Klein AL. Diastolic heart failure: restrictive cardiomyopathy, constrictive pericarditis, and cardiac tamponade: clinical and echocardiographic evaluation. Cardiol Rev 2002;10(4): 218–29.

Management of Common Cardiovascular Emergencies in Critically Ill Patients

Yogamaya Mantha, MD[a], Rakushumimarika Harada, MD[a],
Michinari Hieda, MD, MS, PhD[a,b],*

KEYWORDS

- Heart failure • Cardiogenic shock • Inotropes • Vasopressors • Diuretics • Vasodilators
- Arrhythmia • Hypertensive emergency

KEY POINTS

- This article focuses on acute decompensated heart failure, cardiogenic shock, pulmonary embolism, and hypertensive crisis management in the emergency department and the intensive care unit/critical care unit, which includes the use of inotropes, vasopressors, and antiarrhythmic drugs.
- Treatment of acute decompensated heart failure or cardiogenic shock should be approached systematically and must include symptomatic relief and improvement of morbidity and mortality.
- Inotropic and vasopressor agents increase blood pressure and restore end-organ perfusion in the short term, but high-doses and long-term usage of them may be associated with arrhythmias, increased vasoconstriction and subsequent end-organ damage and thus a net balance should be maintained.
- Cardiac arrhythmias, especially atrial fibrillation, are common in critically ill patients with acute decompensated heart failure and require a careful review of exacerbating and contributing factors in order to tailor management.

INTRODUCTION

Cardiogenic shock is defined as hypotension (systolic blood pressure [BP] less than 90 mm Hg or mean BP 30 mm Hg lower than baseline) that lasts more than 30 minutes as a result of severe reduction of cardiac output (CO), less than 2.2 L/min/m[2], and elevated pulmonary capillary wedge pressure (>18 mm Hg).[1] Critically ill patients not only have reduced myocardial contractility but also impairment of ventricular-arterial coupling, causing dysregulation of systemic vascular resistance (SVR). In other words, cardiogenic shock is a critical condition of inadequate end-organ perfusion. These findings are the hallmarks of the dysfunctional hemodynamics in left ventricular (LV) pump failure. Therefore, it is essential to tailor specific treatments according to individual hemodynamic abnormality. And, it is important to identify how to manage hemodynamics with inotropes in regard to end-organ protection.

Guideline recommendations about inotropes or vasopressors, however, were based on non–higher-evidence levels,[2,3] due to difficulties in accomplishing randomized controlled trials with cardiogenic shock patients. Even several clinical studies demonstrated that inotropes might

Sources of Funding: Dr. Hieda was supported by the American Heart Association Strategically Focused Research Network (14SFRN20600009-03). Dr. Hieda was also supported by American Heart Association post-doctoral fellowship grant (18POST33960092) and the Harry S. Moss Heart Trust.
[a] Department of Internal Medicine, Texas Health Presbyterian Hospital of Dallas, 8200 Walnut Hill Lane, Dallas, TX, 75231, USA; [b] Institute for Exercise and Environmental Medicine, Texas Health Presbyterian Hospital Dallas, University of Texas Southwestern Medical Center, 7232 Greenville Avenue, Dallas, TX 75231, USA
* Corresponding author. 7232 Greenville Avenue, Dallas, TX 75232.
E-mail address: MichinariHieda@texashealth.org

Heart Failure Clin 16 (2020) 153–166
https://doi.org/10.1016/j.hfc.2019.11.001

increase adverse effects and mortality.[4–6] But it is true that appropriate usage of cardiovascular emergency drugs has saved several critical patients by treatment based on pathophysiology or etiology of hemodynamic impairment.[5] Hence, efforts are needed to minimize adverse effects of cardiovascular emergency drugs while achieving the full effect for both heart and end organs. If critically ill patients are persistently hypotensive despite initial inotropes or have worsening multiple end-organ function, additional mechanical circulatory support (MCS) devices should be considered.

The clinical decision, whether to continue treatment with inotropes or to apply additional MCS, is critical while monitoring end-organ function and hemodynamic parameters, such as central venous oxygen saturation (Scvo$_2$ $\geq$70%) and lactic acid ($\leq$2 mmol/L).[7] The Scvo$_2$ is an indicator of the balance of oxygen supply and demand in the systemic circulation and is inversely proportional to the ratio of whole-body oxygen consumption and oxygen supply. The Scvo$_2$ might show normal or high value even in patients with shock, due to oxygen utilization disorder secondary to tissue oxygen metabolism abnormality. Therefore, the Scvo$_2$ needs to be monitored (on average every 2–4 hours) in combination with lactic acid levels for critically ill patients.

TREATMENT OF LOW CARDIAC OUTPUT SYNDROME WITH CARDIOGENIC SHOCK

Heart failure (HF) after acute myocardial infarction (AMI) also can occur due to stunning of the heart or hibernation whereas other causes are due to mechanical complications, such as free wall rupture, ventricular septal rupture, papillary muscle rupture, acute mitral regurgitation, and right ventricular (RV) infarction[8] (**Table 1**). Primary medical management for severe HF, or cardiogenic shock as its consequence, is to improve CO by intravenous (IV) inotropes, vasopressors, and vasodilator support (**Table 2**). Moreover, when using inotropes or vasopressors, careful titration and tapering are extremely important and the lowest dose should be used to plan for the shortest time span.[9]

Dobutamine

Dobutamine is a synthetic catecholamine that acts on α_1-adrenergic, β_1-adrenergic, and β_2-adrenergic receptors.[10] In the cardiac myocytes, the stimulation of β_1 receptor produces a relatively strong, additive inotropic effect and a relatively weak chronotropic effect. In the peripheral vasculature, α_1-agonist effect (vasoconstriction) balances the β_2-agonist effect (vasodilatation). This balance is determined by the dose or concentration of dobutamine. For instance, dobutamine (>3 µg/kg/min) acts on β_1-adrenergic receptors to increase cardiac contractility and thereby increases heart rate.[11,12] Despite its lower chronotropic and vasodilation doses (<2–3 µg/kg/min), dobutamine may significantly increase myocardial oxygen consumption, leading to LV mechanical stress. The effective action of the dobutamine at minimum dose required can be confirmed by monitoring hemodynamic indicators, such as CO, Scvo$_2$ or urine production. There may be few cases in which dobutamine is given to patients who are on β-blocker therapy. Patients on β-blocker therapy might need higher doses of dobutamine or switch to another inotrope, such as milrinone, to obtain therapeutic hemodynamic effects.

Several adverse effects of dobutamine should be considered. Tolerance of the dobutamine can develop after a few days of dobutamine usage, and ventricular arrhythmias can occur at any dose.[13] In addition, there are cases of hypereosinophilic myocarditis reported with long-term treatment with dobutamine.[14]

Milrinone

Milrinone is a widely used inotropic agent and has been in use for approximately 2 decades.[13] As a phosphodiesterase inhibitor, it prevents the breakdown of cAMP, which increases the level of cyclic adenosine monophosphate (cAMP) and calcium entry and ejection into myocytes.[13] This results in increased contractility and myocardial relaxation. Because this mechanism is independent from acting on β receptors, milrinone is preferably used in patients with advanced HF on β-blocker therapy. It also is a systemic vasodilator and, in particular, reduces pulmonary artery pressure. Milrinone causes vasodilation of pulmonary vasculature through the cAMP pathway and thereby reduces RV failure.[15] Milrinone has a theoretic benefit, because it does not increase myocardial oxygen consumption compared with dobutamine.[16] In patients with bloodstream infection, however, milrinone is contraindicated due to its vasodilatory effects, which would be counterintuitive.[17] In comparison with dobutamine, milrinone ideally is not used in patients with chronic kidney disease (estimated glomerular filtration rate, $\leq$45 mL/min/1.73 m^2) because it is renally excreted and has a longer half-life, of 30 hours.[18]

The OPTIME- CHF (Outcomes of a Prospective Trial of Intravenous Milrinone for Exacerbations of Chronic Heart Failure) study demonstrated a positive response of short-term milrinone use in patients with acute decompensated HF (ADHF) without cardiogenic shock and suggested a more

Table 1
Post–myocardial infarction complications

Myocardial Infarction Complications	Risk Factors	Treatment	Routine Medical Contraindications
Cardiogenic shock	AMI; previous history of HF; mechanical complications, such as tamponade, mitral regurgitation, wall rupture; female > male	Inotropes, MCS	β-blockers, ACEi, morphine
HF	Previous history of HF, AMI, valvular disease, family history	Diuretics, ACEi/ARB, ARNi, β-blockers	
Mitral regurgitation	Papillary muscle dysfunction/rupture secondary to AMI (culprit: left coronary artery)	Nitrates, sodium nitroprusside, diuretics, IABP, inotropes, emergent surgery	
LV free wall rupture	First MI, anterior infarction, female > male, age, hypertension, NSAIDs use, recent steroid use	Fluids, inotropes, vasopressors, pericardiocentesis, IABP, percutaneous cardiopulmonary bypass	Diuretics, preload reduction
Ventricular septal rupture	Single vessel disease, first MI, fibrinolytic therapy, extensive myocardial damage	Emergency surgery, inotropes, vasodilators, diuretics, IABP	
LV aneurysm	Late reperfusion therapy	ACEi, anti-ischemic medications for angina, anticoagulation, close observation, aneurysmectomy	
Sustained ventricular tachycardia	Ischemia, electrolyte abnormalities, HF	Immediate defibrillation	
Ventricular fibrillation	Ischemia, electrolyte abnormalities, HF	Immediate defibrillation	
Pericarditis	Fibrinolytic therapy	Aspirin, colchicine, pericardiocentesis, pericardial window	Glucocorticoids, NSAIDs for pain relief
Symptomatic bradycardia, AV nodal blockade	Inferior, posterior MI	Transcutaneous or transvenous temporary pacing, atropine	AVN blocking agents

Most common mechanical complications after myocardial infarction and some routine medical therapies and contraindications.

Abbreviations: ACEi, angiotensin-converting enzyme inhibitor; ARB, angiotensin receptor blocker; ARNi, angiotensin receptor neprilysin inhibitor; AVN, AV node; IABP, intra-aortic balloon pump; MI, myocardial infarction; NSAIDs, nonsteroidal anti-inflammatory drugs.

favorable response in patients, especially those with nonischemic cardiomyopathy compared with ischemic cardiomyopathy.[5] The study did not show, however, any difference in mortality, readmission rate, or duration of hospitalization.[5]

It also showed an increased risk of arrhythmias; thus, it is not used routinely in all patients with acute HF.[5] In the PROMISE (Prospective Randomized Milrinone Survival Evaluation) trial, patients with severe chronic HF and LV dysfunction were

Table 2
Different types of inotropes, vasopressors, and vasodilator therapy

Medication	Receptor Affinity	Dose Range	Adverse Effects
NE	$\alpha_1 > \beta_1$	0.01–3.00 µg/kg/min	Bradycardia, peripheral ischemia, hypertension
Epinephrine	$\alpha_1 = \beta_1 > \beta_2$	0.01–0.10 µg/kg/min Bolus: 1 mg IV every 3–5 min with a max of 0.2 mg/kg	Tachyarrhythmias, diaphoresis, renal vasoconstriction, peripheral vasoconstriction
Vasopressin	V_1 receptors in SMC V_2 receptors in renal collecting duct	0.01–0.10 U/min Bolus: 40.0 IV	Hyponatremia, cardiac ischemia, splanchnic vasoconstriction, hypertension
Dopamine	D_1 and D_2	0.5–20.0 µg/kg/min	Tachycardia, proarrhythmic, severe hypertension (in patients with nonselective β-blockers)
Dobutamine	$\beta_1 > \beta_2$	2.0–20.0 µg/kg/min If needed >10, please consider MCS device.	Ventricular premature contractions, angina pectoris, hypotension
Milrinone	PDEi	0.375–0.75 µg/kg/min Bolus: 50 µg/kg	Vasodilation, torsades de pointes, cardiac ischemia
Levosimendan	Calcium sensitizer	0.05–0.20 µg/kg/min Bolus: 12–24 µg/kg over 10 min	Hypotension, tachycardia
Digoxin	Na^+-K^+ ATPase	Bolus 0.50 mg IV PO/IV 0.25 mg 12 h later	Bradycardia, advanced AV block

Abbreviations: max, maximum; PDEi, phosphodiesterase inhibitor; SMC, smooth muscle cell; V_1, vasopressin$_1$ receptor; V_2, vasopressin$_2$ receptor; α_1, alpha$_1$-adrenergic receptor; β_1, beta$_1$-adrenergic receptor; β_2, beta$_2$-adrenergic receptor.

randomized to oral milrinone or placebo to determine the effect of milrinone on the mortality as their primary endpoint.[19] According to the trial, all patients who were New Year Heart Association functional class III or class IV showed significantly higher mortality and hospitalizations who were treated with milrinone.[19] Milrinone can increase CO and restore end-organ perfusion in the short term, but high-doses and long-term usage of them may be harmful, and thus a net balance should be considered. Meanwhile, amrinone is used less because of its side effects, which include dose-related thrombocytopenia.[13] Some of the concerning side effects include cardiac arrhythmias.

Norepinephrine

Norepinephrine (NE) is a potent vasopressor because it acts on α_1 receptors and β receptors but it has a weaker β-receptor affinity and thus causes increased peripheral vasoconstriction.[20] It increases mean arterial pressure, and does not increase heart rate or myocardial oxygen consumption compared with its counterparts, epinephrine and dopamine.[21,22] For instance, ADHF complicated with sepsis is a good indication for NE. Titration of NE is dependent on several parameters, including adequate urine production, SVR, lactic acidosis, and Scvo$_2$. Oliguria and azotemia from impaired renal blood flow may warrant decrease in NE and addition of another class of medication, such as vasopressin or dobutamine.

Vasopressin

Vasopressin, or antidiuretic hormone (ADH), acts on V_1 (V_{1a} in vascular smooth muscle and V_{1b} in the pituitary gland) and V_2 receptors. V_{1a} stimulation causes constriction of vascular smooth muscle, whereas V_2 receptors mediate water reabsorption by enhancing renal collecting duct permeability.[13] It causes indirect coronary vasoconstriction as vasopressin primary acts on peripheral smooth muscle. Vasopressin therapy, therefore, may be effective in NE-resistant vasodilatory or cardiogenic shock, improving mean BP and cardiac index and reducing the need for higher doses of NE.[23] The use of vasopressin at low to moderate doses may allow decreased use of NE, and it may be particularly useful in settings prolonged critical illness.[13]

Dopamine

Dopamine has classically been used in the management of HF patients who are suffering from acute hypotension. Dobutamine and dopamine have a class IIa recommendation in patients with ST-elevation myocardial infarction and cardiogenic shock.[24] It demonstrates dose-dependent action, primarily on D_1 and D_2 receptors; low doses cause vasodilation in cerebral, cardiac, and renal arteries. Intermediate doses cause an inotropic effect due to the activation of β_2 receptors; higher doses cause peripheral vasoconstriction via activation of α_1 receptors.[20] In patients with AMI plus cardiogenic shock, it was concluded that at present, there are no convincing data of a superior inotropic agent to reduce mortality.[25] Furthermore, among patients with cardiogenic shock, the mortality rate was significantly higher in patients treated with dopamine than that with NE, although it might be expected that CO would be better maintained with dopamine.[20] Despite successful revascularization and inotropes and/or vasopressor support, many patients may continue to deteriorate in a downward spiral.[26] As necessary, the use of MCS should supersede addition or further titration of vasopressors.[1]

Digoxin

Digoxin is a Na^+-K^+ ATPase inhibitor, which causes increased intracellular concentrations of sodium, which, in turn, causes increased levels of calcium through the Na^+-Ca^{2+} channel. It results in increased cardiac contractility.[27] A Digitalis Investigation Goup study demonstrated that digoxin reduced HF hospitalization; there were no favorable effects on mortality.[28] Patients with HF with reduced ejection fraction (HFrEF) and with atrial fibrillation (AF) benefit from the use of digoxin.[27] Digoxin improved neurohormonal profile, including brain natriuretic peptide and/or atrial natriuretic peptide.[29,30] Theoretically, it has shown utility in weaning from IV inotrope therapy because it can be used orally.

Digoxin generally should be avoided in patients with advanced atrioventricular (AV) block, or accessory AV pathways, because it blocks the AV node causing a reduction in atrial rate or increases the risk of bradyarrhythmia. Additionally, it should be used cautiously in patients with renal impairment, hypokalemia, hypomagnesemia, and hypothyroidism in order to prevent digoxin intoxication.[29]

Vasodilators

Vasodilators can be classified as (1) venodilators, (2) arterial dilators, or (3) venoarterial dilators, and they activate guanylate cyclase in the smooth muscle cells, which increases intracellular cyclic guanylate monophosphate resulting in vessel relaxation.[31] In patients with ADHF, especially with abnormal fluid distribution and/or afterload mismatch, immediate decrease in LV preload and afterload is paramount.

Nitroglycerin can be used as the first-line vasodilator agent, with a loading dose of 20 μg/min with a rapid up titration by doubling the dose up to a maximum of 400 μg/min. Sodium nitroprusside, 0.3 μg/min, can be uptitrated to 5 μg/min. Tachyphylaxis, or nitrate tolerance, is common with extended use, usually after 3 days to 4 days. The nitrate tolerance is proposed due to decreased nitroglycerin to nitric oxide, reduced bioactivity of nitric oxide over time, or neurohormonal activation (renin-angiotensin-aldosterone system, which increases sympathetic nervous system).[32] This is initiated by increased vascular superoxide production and a supersensitivity to vasoconstrictors secondary to a tonic activation of protein kinase C.[33] As a result, increased oxidative stress and bioactivation of nitroglycerin contribute to nitroglycerin tolerance.[33] The most effective prevention for the tachyphylaxis is intermittent therapy with an adequate nitrate-free interval (approximately 12 hours), which may restore vascular responsiveness. There are not many cases of cyanide toxicity but it may occur in doses of 250 μg/min for more than 48 hours, especially in patients with hepatic dysfunction, and leads to irreversible neurologic changes and cardiac arrest.

Diuretics

Volume overload, a most common complication of fluid retention, is frequently encountered in an emergency department or intensive care unit. Diuretics are the mainstay treatment of ADHF with pulmonary and peripheral edema and are able to provide rapid symptom relief (**Table 3**). Administered IV, diuretics provide vigorous diuresis, which also may result in adverse effects or diuretic resistance simultaneously. Therefore, it is necessary to be familiar with the half-life and properties of diuretics for appropriate use. Clinicians must consider individual etiologies, comorbidities, and monitor urine production every hour and electrolytes accordingly.

Loop Diuretics

Loops diuretics are the primary pharmacologic treatment of volume overload with ADHF[34]

Table 3
Diuretic therapy for acute decompensated heart failure

Diuretic	Dose	Duration of Action	Management Consideration
Loop			
Furosemide	20–40 mg or 2.5 × outpatient dose Up titrate up to 160 mg 1-time dose or infusion, 5–40 mg/h	6–8 h	IV > PO, monitor electrolytes
Bumetanide	PO: 0.5–1.0 mg, max 10 mg/d IV: 1–4/0.5–2 mg/h (max 2–4 mg/h) Up titrate up to 2–4 mg 1-time dose or infusion	4–6 h	Monitor electrolytes Ventricular tachyarrhythmias due to electrolyte abnormalities is common.
Torsemide	10–20 mg 1-time dose or bolus up to 20–100 mg, IV infusion up to 5–20 mg/h	12–16 h	Adverse effects include ototoxicity
Thiazide			Combination therapy with loop diuretics to counter diuretic resistance
Chlorothiazide	250–500 mg IV or 500–1000 mg PO	6–12 h	Only IV thiazide diuretic
Metolazone	2.5–10 mg PO d	12–24 h	
Hydrochlorothiazide	25–50 mg BID	6–12 h	
Potassium sparing			
Spironolactone	25–50 mg PO d	48–96 h	If hypokalemia
Eplerenone	25–50 mg PO d	48 h	If hypokalemia
Vasopressin V_2-receptor antagonist			Hypernatremia, intravascular dehydration, central pontine myelinolysis
Tolvaptan	15–30 mg PO daily, max 60 mg	NS	If hyponatremia (Na <125 mEq/L)
Satavaptan	25–50 mg PO once	NS	
Conivaptan	20 mg IV loading dose (m followed by 20 mg continuous IV infusion/ day (max 40 mg)	NS	

Abbreviations: max, maximum; NS, not specified.

(**Table 4**). Loop diuretics, including furosemide, bumetanide, and torsemide, act by reversibly inhibiting the Na^+-K^+-$2Cl^-$ symporter (cotransporter) on the apical membrane of epithelial cells in the thick ascending loop of Henle.[35] The efficacy of loop diuretics depends on renal plasma blood flow and proximal tubule secretion to deliver these agents to their site of action.[35]

According to the DOSE (Diuretic Optimization Strategies Evaluation) study, patients with chronic diuretic therapy should receive 2.5 times the outpatient management.[36] One of the limitations of furosemide is its half-life, which is 1.5 hours, compared with that of torsemide, which is 6.3 hours and has better bioavailability.[35,37] In patients with LV pump failure, blood flow to renal vasculature is limited and thus can cause volume overload (>5–10 L) that is refractory to higher doses of loop diuretic therapy.[38] In these cases, a continuous infusion and/or bolus can be considered. In order to

Table 4
Management of clinical situations in acute decompensated heart failure

Clinical Situations	Management Consideration/Comments
Is patient on outpatient diuretics?	First-line agent is furosemide, and consider 2.5 × outpatient dose.
Is patient adequately producing urine on 1 agent?	If initially on IV loop diuretic, consider adding thiazide.
Does patient have any adverse effects of diuretics?	Treat electrolyte abnormalities with repletion and frequent laboratory evaluation and acute hypoxic respiratory failure with oxygen supplementation (Spo_2 <90%), maintain low-sodium diet ($\leq$3 g/d), fluid restriction ($\leq$1.5–2 L), continuous telemetry to monitor for arrhythmias.
Refractory edema	Consider boluses and/or continuous IV loop (furosemide, torsemide, bumetanide) and/or thiazide (IV chlorothiazide) or PO metolazone or hydrochlorothiazide; consider IV albumin or gentle hydration with normal saline; keep diuretic agent in the vascular space. Acetazolamide for contraction metabolic alkalosis (250–500 mg, once or twice a day).
Cardiorenal syndrome	Consider IV infusion with loop diuretics if fluid boluses are insufficient. Treat underlying cause, which is HF, with inotropic agents such as dobutamine that increases forward flow and renal splanchnic vasodilation. Vasodilator therapy with (IV nitroprusside or nitroglycerin) or PO hydralazine to reduce preload. Ultrafiltration to decrease volume overload for refractory cardiorenal syndrome as last resort.
Hypervolemic hyponatremia	Consider treating with vasopressin receptor antagonists for symptomatic hyponatremia (<120 mg/dL). Consider hypertonic saline with high-dose furosemide (250 mg IV BID) to increase creatinine clearance and to keep diuretic in vascular space.
Strategies to decrease morbidity and mortality	β-blockers, ACEi/ARB, ARNi, potassium-sparing diuretics, ivabradine

Abbreviations: ACEi, angiotension-converting enzyme inhibitors; ARB, angiotensin receptor blocker; ARNi, angiotension receptor neprilysin inhibiton.

overcome loop diuretic resistance, combination nephron blockade with thiazide diuretics may be considered. IV chlorothiazide (500–1000 mg) or oral metolazone can be effective but can cause profound electrolyte abnormalities and hypotension, which need to be monitored.[39] Another strategy is to introduce hypertonic saline, to keep the diuretic in the vascular space, which thereby increases the delivery to the kidney. The SMAC-HF (Short-term effects of hypertonic saline solution in acute heart failure and long-term effects of a moderate sodium restriction in patients with compensated heart failure with New York Heart Association class III (Class C)) study demonstrated that IV, 3% saline, with IV furosemide, 250 mg IV twice daily, with moderate Na^+ restriction increased creatinine clearance compared with only IV furosemide and Na^+ restriction.[40]

Potassium-Sparing Diuretics

If profound hypokalemia is observed, potassium-sparing diuretics, such as spironolactone and eplerenone, can be considered. A recent trial showed high-dose spironolactone (100 mg) significantly improved diuresis in patients with ADHF but did not improve 60-day mortality and rehospitalization rate.[41]

Vasopressin Receptor Antagonists

In clinical scenarios, such as ADHF with hyponatremia, vasopressin antagonists are beneficial. Tolvaptan, lixivaptan, and satavaptan are vasopressin receptor antagonists that negate the effects of increased circulated levels of arginine vasopressin.[42] Vasopressin receptor antagonists currently are approved for short-term therapy (<30 days) for symptomatic hyponatremia (Na^+ <125 mEq/L) in patients who are refractory to traditional methods, such as fluid and Na^+ restriction and diuretics.[43] Increased levels of vasopressin lead to increased SVR and positive water balance. These agents interact particularly with V_{1a}, V_{1b}, and V_2 receptors located in the vascular endothelium, anterior pituitary gland, and renal tubular collecting ducts, respectively, and decrease vasopressin activity.[23] The EVEREST (Efficacy of Vasopressin Antagonism in Heart Failure Outcome Study with Tolvaptan) trial investigated short-term and long-term effects of inhibiting arginine vasopressin in patients with symptomatic HF and showed decrease symptoms, such as dyspnea, edema, and body weight, but did not show long-term morbidity and mortality benefit.[42] In addition, the ACTIV (Acute and Chronic Therapeutic Impact of a Vasopressin Antagonist in Congestive Heart Failure) in HF trial showed tolvaptan significantly increased urine production and even normalized Na^+ levels in patients with ADHF.[44] Because adverse effects, such as hypernatremia, intravascular dehydration, and central pontine myelinolysis, may occur with excessive diuresis, water restriction during administration of tolvaptan is contraindicated and can cause deleterious effects.[45,46] Thus, it is necessary to rehydrate orally. It is important to monitor serum Na^+ concentration and urine specific gravity carefully.

PULMONARY EMBOLISM

Acute pulmonary embolism usually originates from lower extremity deep vein thrombosis or venous thromboembolism (VTE). The presentation of PE can be asymptomatic or can present with symptoms of RV HF secondary to acute increase in afterload. PE can be stratified by the clot burden into low-risk, submassive, and massive PE.[47]

Anticoagulation remains the cornerstone of treatment of acute PE. For patients with average bleeding risk, unfractionated heparin should be bolused at 80 U/kg followed by an infusion at 18 U/kg/h. Anti–factor Xa monitoring instead of activated partial thromboplastin time is more popular in the clinical setting because it measures heparin directly.[48] Low-molecular-weight heparin (LMWH) is an alternative therapy to unfractionated heparin and has greater bioavailability and longer half-life, thus does not require coagulation profile monitoring.[48]

Fondaparinux directly inhibitors factor X. It has a fixed dose and us used once daily subcutaneously. Because LMWH and fondaparinux are metabolized by the kidney, patients with renal insufficiency require renal dosing. Bridging with LMWH is necessary, especially for direct oral anticoagulant, such as warfarin. The BRIDGE (Perioperative Bridging Anticoagulation in Patients with Atrial Fibrillation) trial demonstrated that in patients with AF, bridging with LMWH had increased risk of major bleeding compared with nonbridged patients.[49] Routine bridging is still seen, however, in clinical practice. On the contrary, novel oral anticoagulants do not require bridging or coagulation profile monitoring.[50]

Two other modalities of treatment include fibrinolysis and surgical intervention.[51] The PEITHO (Pulmonary Embolism Thrombolysis) trial concluded that in patients with intermediate-risk or submassive PE, fibrinolytic therapy prevented hemodynamic decompensation with subsequent risk of major hemorrhage and stroke.[52] Patients with submassive or massive PE who exhibit hemodynamic compromise warrant immediate advanced therapy, including fibrinolysis.[52]

ARRHYTHMIAS

Arrhythmias are common in critically ill patients. Longstanding refractory arrhythmias can cause heart remodeling, leading to HF; thus, rate control must be used to prevent ultrastructural changes.[6] The limiting factor for the medications is the associated adverse effects due to dose-dependent and dose-independent toxicities (**Table 5**). For hemodynamically unstable patients, immediate cardioversion is recommended. In addition to stabilizing hemodynamics, treating the underlying cause, such as hypoxemia, hypotension, acid-base, or electrolyte abnormality, is essential. Because arrhythmias are a vast topic, the authors focused more on relatively the most common arrhythmia, AF, associated with ADHF.

AF during AMI is associated with increased mortality and chances of stroke particularly in anterior infarction.[53] Pharmacologic cardioversion with either ibutilide or amiodarone is recommended if patients are not indicated for immediate cardioversion.[54] Dofetilide and amiodarone are

Table 5
Acute management of arrhythmias

Type of Arrhythmia	Medication	Dose	Comments
AF/atrial flutter			More than 50% of episodes convert spontaneously; correct underlying HF, stress, pain, and or electrolyte abnormalities first.
Rate Control	β-blockers		Rule out WPW syndrome first.
	Metoprolol	2.5–5 mg IV over 2–5 min	Up to 15 mg in 15 min
	Esmolol	0.5 mg/kg IV over 1 min, then IV drip 50–200 mg/kg/min	
	Ca^{2+} channel blockers		Patients who cannot tolerate β-blockers Avoided in patients with HFrEF due to their negative inotropic effects
	Diltiazem	0.25 mg/kg IV over 2 min, then IV drip 5–15 mg/h	Contraindicated in hypotension due to LV dysfunction
	Verapamil	0.075–0.15 mg/kg IV over 2 min	Contraindicated in hypotension due to LV dysfunction
Rhythm control/pharmacologic cardioversion			
	Digoxin	0.25 mg IV every 2 h (up to 1.5 mg in 24 h)	Benefits patients with HFrEF and HFpEF
	Amiodarone	150 mg IV over 10 min, then IV drip 1 mg/min for 6 h followed by 0.5 mg/min for 18 h (total 1.05 g over 24 h)	Long half-life of amiodarone (25–100 d) Multiple side effects; lung, liver, thyroid, and kidney dysfunction Careful monitoring, including the drug concentration, thyroid and liver functions, and chest radiograph
	Ibutilide	1 mg IV over 10 min	QTc prolongation and increase the risk of torsades de pointes, especially in patients with HF
AF with preexcitation or WPW	Procainamide	15–18 mg/kg over 25–30 min or 100 mg given no faster than 50 mg/min, may repeat every 5 min (max cumulative dose 1 g); then IV drip 1–4 mg/min	
	Ibutilide	1 mg IV over 10 min	
Wide complex tachycardia	Amiodarone	150 mg IV over 10 min, may repeat every 10 min as needed; then IV drip 1 mg/min for 6 h, followed by 0.5 mg/min for 18 h (max cumulative dose 2.2 g over 24 h)	Can cause VT, torsades de pointes, HFpEF exacerbation, hypotension

(continued on next page)

Table 5
(continued)

Type of Arrhythmia	Medication	Dose	Comments
	Procainamide	Same dosage as AF with pre-excitation or WPW	
	Lidocaine	1–1.5 mg/kg IV, may repeat 0.5–0.75 mg/kg every 5–10 min (max cumulative dose 3 mg/kg); then IV drip 1–4 mg/min	
Supraventricular tachycardia	Adenosine	6 mg followed 20 mL NS bolus, wait 1–2 min, 12 mg followed by 20 mL NS bolus (max 12 mg)	Therapeutic and diagnostic as adenosine terminates AV nodal dependent SVT, such as AVNRT and AVRT and will unmask atrial tachycardia, such as atrial flutter/fibrillation.

Abbreviations: AVNRT, atrioventricular nodal reentrant tachycardia; AVRT, atrioventricular reentrant tachycardia; HFpEF, HF with preserved ejection fraction; max, maximum; NS, normal saline; QTc, corrected QT time; SVT, sustained ventricular tachycardia; VT, ventricular tachycardia; WPW, Wolff-Parkinson-White syndrome.

the only guideline-recommended antiarrhythmic drugs for the treatment of AF in patients with HF but they are not without side effects, which include prolongation of QT interval and torsades de pointes.[55] Amiodarone is preferred in patients with HFrEF because it can slow ventricular rate via β-blockade and Ca^{2+} channel blockade.[54] In critically ill patients with AF, 150-mg IV bolus of amiodarone over 10 minutes is recommended (if necessary, bolus may be repeated in 10–30 min); then, 1 mg per minute for 6 hours; and then, 0.5 mg per minute for 18 hours, which then can be reduced or converted to oral dosing when possible.[56] For the potential adverse effects, careful monitoring, including the serum drug concentration, thyroid and liver functions, and chest radiograph, is essential for patients taking amiodarone (see **Table 5**).

HYPERTENSIVE CRISIS

Hypertensive crises can be stratified into (1) hypertensive emergency, which includes the presence of acute end-organ damage, or (2) hypertensive urgency, which has an absence of acute target organ damage. Generally, both present with significantly elevated BP (systolic BP ≥180 mm Hg and/or diastolic BP ≥120 mm Hg).[57] Patients with chronic hypertension may present with severe hypertension, which is defined as BP of 180/110 mm Hg to 220/130 mm Hg without end-organ damage and these patients usually tolerate higher BPs.[58] Target organ damage can be defined as the

acute damage and resulting in acute coronary syndrome, acute ischemic or hemorrhagic stroke, posterior leukoencephalopathy syndrome, retinopathy, acute renal insufficiency, aortic dissection, or pulmonary edema.[59] Overall, hypertensive emergency must be rapidly recognized and the reduction in BP by 10% to 20% during the first hour should be achieved by IV antihypertensive medications. Some conditions, such as aortic dissection, require rapid decrease of systolic BP with usually a target to less than 140 mm Hg in the first hour.[59]

Pharmacologic interventions include IV β-blockers, Ca^{2+} channel blockers, and vasodilators but selection of each antihypertensive requires careful review of etiology, degree of progression of target organ damage, the desired rate of decrease in BP, and comorbidities[59] (**Table 6**). IV labetalol, a combined α-blocker and β-blocker, and nicardipine, are the 2 most commonly used in clinical practice. Labetalol usually has a longer half-life than nicardipine or nitroprusside and may cause systemic hypotension which should be avoided. β-blockers generally are contraindicated in acute pulmonary edema, reactive airway disease, bradycardia, and advanced heart block AMI. Nicardipine has a relatively shorter half-life and comparatively is shown to have a more predictable reduction of BP.[60] Vasodilators frequently are used for hypertensive crises, which include hydralazine, nitroprusside, and nitroglycerin. Generally, nitroglycerin is used in patients with acute coronary syndrome only after β-blocker administration to prevent reflex tachycardia. Moreover,

Table 6
Management of hypertensive emergency according to comorbidities

Clinical Scenario	Preferred Drug	Usual Dose	Rate of Blood Pressure Decline	Comments
Posterior leukoencephalopathy syndrome	Labetalol	10–20 mg IV push over 2 min; 0.5–2 mg/min	Immediate MAP reduction to 20%–25%	
Aortic dissection	Esmolol	500–1000 µg/kg over 1 min; 50 µg/kg/min infusion (max 200 µg/kg/min)	Immediate, keep systemic BP <120 mm Hg	Prevent reflex tachycardia
	Labetalol	10–20 mg IV push over 2 min; 0.5–2 mg/min		
Acute coronary syndrome	Metoprolol	5 mg IV; every 5 min up to 3 doses; max 15 mg	Immediate, keep MAP between 60 mm Hg and 100 mm Hg.	Nitroprusside should be avoided in coronary steal syndrome. β-blockers should be avoided in bradycardia, second- or third-degree heart block and reactive airway disease.
	Labetalol	10–20 mg IV push over 2 min; 0.5–2 mg/min		
	Nitroglycerin	5–20 µg/min, increase 5 µg/min every 5 min		
Acute pulmonary edema	Nitroglycerin with loop diuretic	5–20 µg/min, increase 5 µg/min every 5 min	Immediate, keep MAP between 60 mm Hg and 100 mm Hg.	β-blockers are contraindicated.
Acute renal failure	Labetalol	10–20 mg IV push over 2 min; 0.5–2 mg/min	Decrease MAP 20%–25% over the first 12 h.	Avoid ACEi in acute phase.
	Nitroprusside	0.3–0.5 µg/kg/min, increase by 0.5 µg/kg/min (max 2 µg/kg/min		
Intracranial hemorrhage	Labetalol	10–20 mg IV push over 2 min; 0.5–2 mg/min	Decrease systolic BP <180 mm Hg within the first h.	
	Nicardipine	5 mg/h; titrate by 2.5 mg/h every 5 to 15 min (max 15 mg/h)		
Ischemic stroke	Labetalol	10–20 mg IV push over 2 min; 0.5–2 mg/min	Decrease MAP by 15% in the first h.	
Retinopathy	Labetalol	10–20 mg IV push over 2 min; 0.5–2 mg/min	Decrease MAP 20%–25% over the first 12 h.	

Abbreviations: ACEi, angiotensin-converting enzyme inhibitor; h, hour; MAP, mean arterial pressure; min, minutes.

patients with LV dysfunction secondary to hypertensive emergency may present with acute HF. In such cases, nitroprusside with concomitant use of loop diuretics are used to lower SVR and decrease acute pulmonary edema, which further lowers the BP.[58] On the contrary, nitroprusside generally is contraindicated in patients with AMI because it causes coronary steal syndrome, which extends the infarction.[61]

SUMMARY

The etiology of HF or cardiogenic shock is important for management of patients in the critical care setting. ADHF most often encompasses a complex and heterogeneous group of syndromes covering multiple disease states with diverse presentations. It is paramount to minimize adverse effects of inotropes and vasopressors while achieving the full effect for both heart and end organs. Clinicians should aim to lower complications by choosing medications with respect to comorbidities and close the gap between evidence-based medicine and clinical practice.

ACKNOWLEDGMENTS

We appreciate Toler Freyaldenhoven and Yi-Jin Hsieh for dedicating time and effort for proofreading this article.

DISCLOSURE

The authors have nothing to disclose.

CONFLICT OF INTEREST

None.

REFERENCES

1. Shah P, Cowger JA. Cardiogenic shock. Crit Care Clin 2014;30(3):391–412.
2. Steg PG, James SK, Atar D, et al. ESC Guidelines for the management of acute myocardial infarction in patients presenting with ST-segment elevation. Eur Heart J 2012;33(20):2569–619.
3. O'Gara PT, Kushner FG, Ascheim DD, et al. 2013 ACCF/AHA guideline for the management of ST-elevation myocardial infarction: executive summary: a report of the American College of Cardiology Foundation/American Heart Association Task Force on Practice Guidelines. Circulation 2013;127(4): 529–55.
4. Francis GS, Bartos JA, Adatya S. Inotropes. J Am Coll Cardiol 2014;63(20):2069–78.
5. Felker GM, Benza RL, Chandler AB, et al. Heart failure etiology and response to milrinone in decompensated heart failure: results from the OPTIME-CHF study. J Am Coll Cardiol 2003;41(6): 997–1003.
6. Yancy Clyde W, Jessup M, Bozkurt B, et al. 2013 ACCF/AHA guideline for the management of heart failure. Circulation 2013;128(16):e240–327.
7. Mayer K, Trzeciak S, Puri NK. Assessment of the adequacy of oxygen delivery. Curr Opin Crit Care 2016;22(5):437–43.
8. Werdan K, Russ M, Buerke M, et al. Evidence-based management of cardiogenic shock after acute myocardial infarction. Interv Cardiol 2013;8(2):73–80.
9. Levy B, Buzon J, Kimmoun A. Inotropes and vasopressors use in cardiogenic shock: when, which and how much? Curr Opin Crit Care 2019;25(4): 384–90.
10. Psotka MA, Gottlieb SS, Francis GS, et al. Cardiac calcitropes, myotropes, and mitotropes: JACC review topic of the week. J Am Coll Cardiol 2019; 73(18):2345–53.
11. Coletta AP, Cleland JG, Freemantle N, et al. Clinical trials update from the European Society of Cardiology Heart Failure meeting: SHAPE, BRING-UP 2 VAS, COLA II, FOSIDIAL, BETACAR, CASINO and meta-analysis of cardiac resynchronisation therapy. Eur J Heart Fail 2004;6(5):673–6.
12. Follath F, Cleland JG, Just H, et al. Efficacy and safety of intravenous levosimendan compared with dobutamine in severe low-output heart failure (the LIDO study): a randomised double-blind trial. Lancet 2002;360(9328):196–202.
13. Overgaard CB, Dzavik V. Inotropes and vasopressors: review of physiology and clinical use in cardiovascular disease. Circulation 2008;118(10):1047–56.
14. Ginsberg F, Parrillo JE. Eosinophilic myocarditis. Heart Fail Clin 2005;1(3):419–29.
15. Ginwalla M, Tofovic DS. Current status of inotropes in heart failure. Heart Fail Clin 2018;14(4):601–16.
16. Grose R, Strain J, Greenberg M, et al. Systemic and coronary effects of intravenous milrinone and dobutamine in congestive heart failure. J Am Coll Cardiol 1986;7(5):1107–13.
17. Kohsaka S, Menon V, Lowe AM, et al. Systemic inflammatory response syndrome after acute myocardial infarction complicated by cardiogenic shock. Arch Intern Med 2005;165(14):1643–50.
18. Cox ZL, Calcutt MW, Morrison TB, et al. Elevation of plasma milrinone concentrations in stage D heart failure associated with renal dysfunction. J Cardiovasc Pharmacol Ther 2013;18(5):433–8.
19. Packer M, Carver JR, Rodeheffer RJ, et al. Effect of oral milrinone on mortality in severe chronic heart failure. The PROMISE Study Research Group. N Engl J Med 1991;325(21):1468–75.
20. De Backer D, Biston P, Devriendt J, et al. Comparison of dopamine and norepinephrine in the treatment of shock. N Engl J Med 2010;362(9):779–89.

21. Unverzagt S, Wachsmuth L, Hirsch K, et al. Inotropic agents and vasodilator strategies for acute myocardial infarction complicated by cardiogenic shock or low cardiac output syndrome. Cochrane Database Syst Rev 2014;(1):CD009669.

22. Levy B, Clere-Jehl R, Legras A, et al. Epinephrine versus norepinephrine for cardiogenic shock after acute myocardial infarction. J Am Coll Cardiol 2018;72(2):173–82.

23. Dunser MW, Mayr AJ, Ulmer H, et al. Arginine vasopressin in advanced vasodilatory shock: a prospective, randomized, controlled study. Circulation 2003; 107(18):2313–9.

24. Werdan K, Russ M, Buerke M, et al. Cardiogenic shock due to myocardial infarction: diagnosis, monitoring and treatment: a German-Austrian S3 Guideline. Dtsch Arztebl Int 2012;109(19):343–51.

25. Schumann J, Henrich EC, Strobl H, et al. Inotropic agents and vasodilator strategies for the treatment of cardiogenic shock or low cardiac output syndrome. Cochrane Database Syst Rev 2018;1:CD009669.

26. Džavík V, Lawler PR. Unloading is not the only question in cardiogenic shock. J Am Coll Cardiol 2019; 73(6):663.

27. Eichhorn EJ, Gheorghiade M. Digoxin. Prog Cardiovasc Dis 2002;44(4):251–66.

28. Digitalis Investigation Group. The effect of digoxin on mortality and morbidity in patients with heart failure. N Engl J Med 1997;336(8):525–33.

29. Gheorghiade M, van Veldhuisen Dirk J, Colucci Wilson S. Contemporary use of digoxin in the management of cardiovascular disorders. Circulation 2006;113(21):2556–64.

30. Newton GE, Tong JH, Schofield AM, et al. Digoxin reduces cardiac sympathetic activity in severe congestive heart failure. J Am Coll Cardiol 1996; 28(1):155–61.

31. Daiber A, Münzel T. Organic nitrate therapy, nitrate tolerance, and nitrate-induced endothelial dysfunction: emphasis on redox biology and oxidative stress. Antioxid Redox Signal 2015;23(11):899–942.

32. Parker JD, Parker JO. Nitrate therapy for stable angina pectoris. N Engl J Med 1998;338(8):520–31.

33. Munzel T, Daiber A, Mulsch A. Explaining the phenomenon of nitrate tolerance. Circ Res 2005;97(7): 618–28.

34. Bergethon KE, Ju C, DeVore AD, et al. Trends in 30-day readmission rates for patients hospitalized with heart failure: findings from the get with the guidelines-heart failure registry. Circ Heart Fail 2016;9(6) [pii:e002594].

35. Jentzer JC, DeWald TA, Hernandez AF. Combination of loop diuretics with thiazide-type diuretics in heart failure. J Am Coll Cardiol 2010;56(19):1527–34.

36. Felker GM, Lee KL, Bull DA, et al. Diuretic strategies in patients with acute decompensated heart failure. N Engl J Med 2011;364(9):797–805.

37. Vargo DL, Kramer WG, Black PK, et al. Bioavailability, pharmacokinetics, and pharmacodynamics of torsemide and furosemide in patients with congestive heart failure. Clin Pharmacol Ther 1995; 57(6):601–9.

38. Koniari K, Parissis J, Paraskevaidis I, Anastasiou-Nana M. Treating volume overload in acutely decompensated heart failure: established and novel therapeutic approaches. Eur Heart J Acute Cardiovasc Care 2012;1(3):256–68.

39. Fliser D, Schroter M, Neubeck M, et al. Coadministration of thiazides increases the efficacy of loop diuretics even in patients with advanced renal failure. Kidney Int 1994;46(2):482–8.

40. Paterna S, Fasullo S, Parrinello G, et al. Short-term effects of hypertonic saline solution in acute heart failure and long-term effects of a moderate sodium restriction in patients with compensated heart failure with New York Heart Association class III (Class C) (SMAC-HF Study). Am J Med Sci 2011;342(1): 27–37.

41. Apriansyah FP, Hersunarti N, Hanafy DA. High-dose spironolactone in high risk acute decompensated heart failure: randomized clinical trial. J Am Coll Cardiol 2019;73(9 Supplement 1):2128.

42. Konstam MA, Gheorghiade M, Burnett JC, et al. Effects of oral tolvaptan in patients hospitalized for worsening heart failure: the EVEREST outcome trial. JAMA 2007;297(12):1319–31.

43. Felker GM, Mentz Robert J, Adams Kirkwood F, et al. Tolvaptan in patients hospitalized with acute heart failure. Circ Heart Fail 2015;8(5):997–1005.

44. Gheorghiade M, Gattis WA, O'Connor CM, et al. Effects of Tolvaptan, a Vasopressin antagonist, in patients hospitalized with worsening heart failurea randomized controlled trial. JAMA 2004;291(16): 1963–71.

45. De Vecchis R, Esposito C, Ariano C, et al. Hypertonic saline plus i.v. furosemide improve renal safety profile and clinical outcomes in acute decompensated heart failure: a meta-analysis of the literature. Herz 2015;40(3):423–35.

46. Gunderson EG, Lillyblad MP, Fine M, et al. Tolvaptan for volume management in heart failure. Pharmacotherapy 2019;39(4):473–85.

47. Busse LW, Vourlekis JS. Submassive pulmonary embolism. Crit Care Clin 2014;30(3):447–73.

48. Garcia DA, Baglin TP, Weitz JI, et al. Parenteral anticoagulants: antithrombotic therapy and prevention of thrombosis, 9th ed: American College of Chest Physicians evidence-based clinical practice guidelines. Chest 2012;141(2 Suppl):e24S–43S.

49. Douketis JD, Spyropoulos AC, Kaatz S, et al. Perioperative bridging anticoagulation in patients with atrial fibrillation. N Engl J Med 2015;373(9):823–33.

50. Raval AN, Cigarroa JE, Chung MK, et al. Management of patients on non-vitamin K antagonist oral

anticoagulants in the acute care and periprocedural setting: a scientific statement from the American Heart Association. Circulation 2017;135(10): e604–33.

51. Piazza G, Goldhaber SZ. Management of submassive pulmonary embolism. Circulation 2010; 122(11):1124–9.

52. Meyer G, Vicaut E, Danays T, et al. Fibrinolysis for patients with intermediate-risk pulmonary embolism. N Engl J Med 2014;370(15):1402–11.

53. Kundu A, O'Day K, Shaikh AY, et al. Relation of atrial fibrillation in acute myocardial infarction to in-hospital complications and early hospital readmission. Am J Cardiol 2016;117(8):1213–8.

54. Tracy C, Boushahri A. Managing arrhythmias in the intensive care unit. Crit Care Clin 2014;30(3): 365–90.

55. January CT, Wann LS, Alpert JS, et al. 2014 AHA/ ACC/HRS guideline for the management of patients with atrial fibrillation: a report of the American College of Cardiology/American Heart Association Task Force on Practice Guidelines and the Heart Rhythm Society. J Am Coll Cardiol 2014;64(21): e1–76.

56. Kusumoto FM, Bailey KR, Chaouki AS, et al. Systematic review for the 2017 AHA/ACC/HRS guideline for management of patients with ventricular arrhythmias and the prevention of sudden cardiac death: a report of the American College of Cardiology/American Heart Association Task Force on Clinical Practice Guidelines and the Heart Rhythm Society. J Am Coll Cardiol 2018;72(14):1653–76.

57. Haddadin F, Munoz Estrella A, Herzog E. Hypertensive emergency presenting with acute spontaneous subdural hematoma. J Cardiol cases 2018;19(1): 25–8.

58. Peixoto AJ. Acute Severe Hypertension. New England Journal of Medicine 2019;381(19):1843–52.

59. Whelton PK, Carey RM, Aronow WS, et al. 2017 ACC/ AHA/AAPA/ABC/ACPM/AGS/APhA/ASH/ASPC/NMA/ PCNA guideline for the prevention, detection, evaluation, and management of high blood pressure in Adults. J Am Coll Cardiol 2018;71(19):e127.

60. Peacock WFIV, Hilleman DE, Levy PD, et al. A systematic review of nicardipine vs labetalol for the management of hypertensive crises. Am J Emerg Med 2012;30(6):981–93.

61. Ihlen H, Myhre E, Opstad P. Evaluation of potential adverse effects of sodium nitroprusside during pacing-induced myocardial ischaemia in man. Eur Heart J 1984;5(10):834–41.

Echocardiography Tips in the Emergency Room

Masataka Sugahara, MD, PhD, Tohru Masuyama, MD, PhD*

KEYWORDS

- Echocardiography • Emergency room • Lung ultrasound • Hemodynamics
- Doppler echocardiography

KEY POINTS

- Acute heart failure is diagnosed by a comprehensive approach, including echocardiography in the emergency room.
- Echocardiography can play an important role in providing instant and relevant information for the effective management of patients with acute heart failure in the emergency room.
- Further investigations by advanced echocardiographic techniques and technologies are expected to improve the initial management and outcomes of patients with acute heart failure in the emergency room.

Heart failure (HF) remains a global health problem because of its high prevalence, readmission rate, and mortality.[1] Of patients with newly diagnosed acute HF (AHF), 80% are admitted via the emergency room (ER) because of acute decompensation.[2] Clinical manifestations with history and physical findings are essential in the diagnosis of AHF. The European Society of Cardiology recommends an algorithmic approach to diagnose and construct therapeutic strategy[3]: the first step is obtaining a clinical history, the second step is performing a physical examination, and the third step is assessing the electrocardiogram and natriuretic peptides. Echocardiography is the fourth step to determine HF etiologies. Mebazaa and colleagues[4] recommend the algorithmic approach with target timeslots (**Fig. 1**). In the flow chart, echocardiographic study is one of the diagnostic components to be performed within 75 minutes of admission to the ER. Therefore, observers (cardiologists in ER or emergency physicians) have to complete the echocardiographic study precisely and determine diagnostic strategy expeditiously. Although the determination of an initial diagnosis is vital for prompt therapeutic attempt in ER, the echocardiographic study may be occasionally restricted because of the patients' status (cardiogenic shock, orthopnea, chest pain, and lung diseases, such as chronic obstructive disease). Otherwise, the echocardiographic study often may not be performed by an experienced cardiologist, but by emergency doctors, anesthesiologists, general practitioners, fellows in training, or experienced sonographers; it is not recommended that fellows and sonographers perform an echocardiographic study without supervision.[5] Therefore, this article aims to enhance the management of AHF by providing echocardiographic tips for emergent settings and outlining critical hemodynamic assessments to be performed in the ER.

ECHOCARDIOGRAPHY IN THE EMERGENT SETTINGS

Patients with AHF may present with emergent or life-threatening status owing to acute coronary syndrome and/or cardiogenic shock. Cardiologists in the ER or emergency physicians are required to assess the current condition and construct a therapeutic strategy in a limited time. Pocket-sized echocardiography is sometimes

JCHO Hoshigaoka Medical Center, 4-8-1 Hoshigaoka, Hirakata, Osaka 573-8511, Japan
* Corresponding author.
E-mail address: tmasuyama-circ@umin.ac.jp

Heart Failure Clin 16 (2020) 167–175
https://doi.org/10.1016/j.hfc.2019.12.003
1551-7136/20/© 2019 Elsevier Inc. All rights reserved.

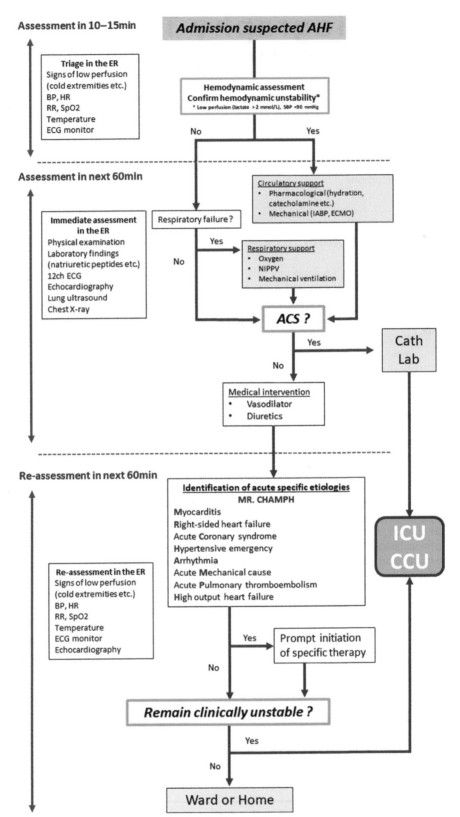

Fig. 1. Algorithmic approach of initial assessment and treatment in patients with suspected AHF. ACS, acute coronary syndrome; BP, blood pressure; CCU, coronary care unit; ECG, electrocardiogram; ECMO, extracorporeal membrane oxygenation; HR, heart rate; IABP, intra-aortic balloon pumping; ICU, intensive care unit; NIPPV, noninvasive positive pressure ventilation; RR, respiratory rate; SBP, systolic BP; SpO₂, peripheral capillary oxygen saturation.

used for the first touch seeking of cardiovascular emergencies owing to take swift action. Therefore, the scope of echocardiography should be focused, and the results should be evaluated intuitively with a conventional technique. In this setting, it may be crucial to assess pericardial effusion, cardiac tamponade, pleural effusion, lung ultrasound (LUS) examinations, global morphologic approaches, wall motion abnormalities, valvular complications, and the inferior vena cava (IVC).

Pericardial Effusion and Cardiac Tamponade

Cardiac tamponade shows hemodynamic alteration by the accumulation of pericardial effusion. Cardiac tamponade is mostly caused by pericarditis (infection, malignancy, autoimmune disease, etc), myocardial rupture owing to acute myocardial infarction or Takotsubo cardiomyopathy, aortic dissection, trauma, renal failure, and hypothyroidism.[6] Echocardiography provides a reliable way of detecting hemodynamic alterations, such as the collapse of the right atrium and right ventricle owing to an increased intrapericardial pressure (**Fig. 2**). Increased pericardial effusion is likely to cause cardiac tamponade; in acute settings, a small amount of pericardial effusion may cause cardiac tamponade. It is difficult to assess cardiac tamponade in patients with mechanical ventilation or a localized defect of the pericardium on Doppler echocardiography. Therefore, simple diagnose by 2-dimensional or M-mode echocardiography is important. Chamber collapse is definitely associated with lowered cardiac output. A short axis view and/or an apical 4-chamber view are useful to detect pericardial effusion and chamber collapsibility.

Pleural Effusion

Accumulation of pleural effusion is one of the physical signs of HF. A large amount of pleural effusion can cause hypoxia and dyspnea. However, the detection of pleural effusion is not robust in HF[7] because its cause is usually multifactorial.

Lung Ultrasound Examination

Visualization of pulmonary congestion by LUS examinations may be useful as a semiquantitative assessment of HF and is recommended as a point-of-focus tool for HF in the ER, although LUS examination may not be categorized as echocardiography. LUS examination is a quick assessment tool and has good intraobserver and interobserver variability.[8] B-lines by LUS examination are longitudinal artifacts that originate from water-thickened interlobular septa and attenuate broadly toward the bottom (the shape is like a comet). It is useful to count the number of B-lines as a diagnostic tool of HF and the number may be used to distinguish HF from lung diseases.[9,10] Pulmonary edema can be suspected by detection of more than 3 B-lines in a rib space in at least 2 scan zones of bilateral side. Although scanning from 8 or more anterior and lateral thoracic zones has been recommended from European Society of Intensive Care Medicine,[11] scanning 6 thoracic regions represented a diagnostic usefulness in the setting of AHF in a multicenter study. Three or more B-lines in 2 or more of 3 bilateral intercostal spaces (6 total views) had high diagnostic usefulness in AHF (**Fig. 3**), and an additive diagnostic usefulness to chest radiography and natriuretic peptides.[8]

Global Morphologic Approach

Assessment of ventricular function is one of the fundamental approaches for hemodynamic assessment. Measurements of left ventricular (LV) volume and the ejection fraction (EF) have been established as a diagnostic and stratifying

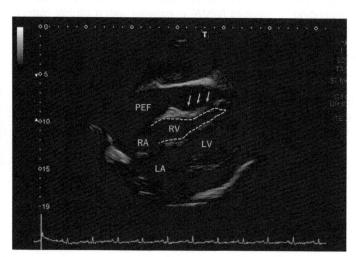

Fig. 2. Echocardiographic feature of cardiac tamponade (etiology: metastatic lung cancer). B-mode echocardiography from subcostal approach showed that RV free wall was compressed by increased intrapericardial pressure in early diastolic phase (*arrows*). LA, left atrium; PEF, pericardial effusion; RA, right atrium.

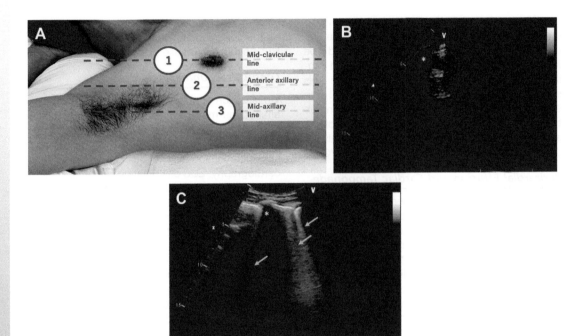

Fig. 3. Evaluation of lung ultrasonography. (*A*) Six scans from left and right anterior chest wall can be useful for LUS examinations. The first zone was located in the second intercostal space on the mid-clavicular line. The second zone was located in the fourth intercostal space on the anterior axillary line. The third zone was located in the fifth intercostal space on the mid-axillary line. (*B*) B-mode echocardiographic image from anterior chest wall showed normal lung. (*C*) B-mode echocardiographic image from anterior chest wall showed that B-lines was visualized from the pleural line (*arrows*). The asterisk marks an acoustic shadow from a rib bone.

tool in HF. Measuring the linear diameter and/or tracing the endocardium is crucial for the determination of chamber volumes. However, measuring chamber volumes may not be practical in emergent settings because these parameters may be inaccurate owing to image quality and volume status at that time.[12] Moreover, measurement of the EF is not essential for the detection of AHF based on Framingham criteria, and eyeball EF is often enough for clinical use. Acute management and initial treatment in the ER do not differ depending on the EF value. Atrial and ventricular sizes are helpful for the recognition of cause and chronicity. An apical 4-chamber view may be useful for understanding global information: biventricular dilatation, ventricular hypertrophy, biatrial dilatation, and so on. In cases of acute right ventricular (RV) failure, RV dilatation causes in a decrease in RV output, compression of interventricular septum toward the LV chamber, a shrinking LV chamber, and a decrease in LV output (**Fig. 4**). Evaluation of RV function by echocardiography is often limited by complex morphology of the right ventricle. Tricuspid annular plane systolic excursion (TAPSE) provides a simple indicative parameter for RV systolic function by M-mode echocardiography. A reduced TAPSE reflects a

deterioration of RV function and is associated with an adverse outcome in patients with pulmonary hypertension, acute decompensation of advanced chronic HF, and other pathophysiology of HF.[13–17]

Wall Motion Abnormality

Echocardiography is one of the most essential methods for the detection of wall motion abnormalities (WMA) in patients with a clinical history, physical examination, and electrocardiogram of acute coronary syndrome in emergency settings. It should be promptly performed to avoid a delay in the transfer to catheter laboratory by cardiologists in the ER or emergency physicians. To assess LV WMA, semiquantitative scoring may be commonly used with the 16- or the 17-segmental model of the American Society of Echocardiography.[18] The scoring is classified as follows: (1) normal or hyperkinesis (normal or hyper wall thickening), (2) hypokinesis (reduced wall thickening), (3) akinesis (absence of wall thickening), or (4) dyskinesis (systolic stretching).

The segmental models are constructed from conventional parasternal views and apical views. When observers suspect acute coronary

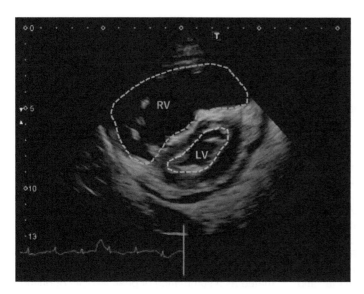

Fig. 4. Evaluation of ventricular interaction from parasternal short axis view. Parasternal short axis view in a patient with worsening pulmonary hypertension owing to connective tissue disease showed that the right ventricle was extensively enlarged by elevated RV systolic pressure (*dotted light blue line*) and left ventricle was compressed via interventricular septum owing to a right ventricular pressure overload (*dotted orange line*).

syndrome, regions of WMA can be predicted from the distribution of culprit and territory of coronary arteries. It should be appreciated that image quality needs to be guaranteed against a loss of assessment; however, the observers may encounter technical difficulties owing to restrictions in the facility, patient complications, or observer skill. Microbubble contrast echocardiography may be an adjunct tool for good visualization of endocardial surface or detection of intracardiac masses in such conditions.[19] Whereas WMA is affected by ventricular conductance abnormalities, including artificial pacing, ventricular interaction, and tissue substrates including scar burden, WMA assessment may be difficult even for experienced observers. Assessment of RV WMA should not be forgotten. Impairment of the RV WMA implies the presence of RV infarction and is a predictive marker for inferior myocardial infarction.[20]

Inferior Vena Cava

Respiratory distensibility of the IVC is one of the indicative parameters for central venous pressure (described in detail in Elevation of Pulmonary Artery Hemodynamics). In the emergent setting, we should pay attention to IVC assessment under intubation with positive pressure ventilation. Positive pressure ventilation influences the central venous pressure.

Acute Mechanical Cause Including Valvular Complications

AHF owing to acute mechanical causes in emergency settings are often perceived as newly emerged systolic or diastolic murmurs that are caused by a rupture of the myocardial wall, disruption of the valvular or arterial apparatus (including infective endocarditis, aortic dissection), or prosthetic valve complication owing to thrombus or dehiscence.

ECHOCARDIOGRAPHY FOR HEMODYNAMIC ASSESSMENT IN THE EMERGENCY ROOM

Evaluation of hemodynamics is crucial in the management of patients with AHF. In clinical guidelines for the management of AHF, routine invasive hemodynamic assessment is recommended only in unstable patients. Therefore, noninvasive hemodynamic assessment by echocardiography is often practical. Doppler echocardiography in particular reflects the real-time behavior of hemodynamics. The Heart Failure Association recommends 3 steps for the assessment in patients with dyspnea in the ER: (1) LUS examination to assess for pulmonary congestion, (2) distensibility of the IVC, and (3) Doppler echocardiography for LV filling pressure. Thus, hemodynamic assessment by Doppler echocardiography is not considered a first-line intervention in the ER.[21]

Elevation of Left Atrial Pressure

Elevation of the left atrial pressure causes pulmonary congestion, and in turn dyspnea. The left atrial pressure has been measured by an invasive method with pulmonary artery catheter; thus, serial assessment of hemodynamic is not practical over days or weeks. A ratio of the peak of early diastolic transmitral flow velocity (E) to the early diastolic mitral annular velocity (E′) has been historically used as a surrogate marker of LV filling pressure,[22] but its use is limited in patients with severe LV dysfunction, significant mitral regurgitation, coronary artery disease, or constrictive pericarditis. Thus, methods for assessing parameters for the detection of elevation left atrial pressure depend on LVEF in the recent guideline from the American Society of Echocardiography.[23] In patients with a preserved EF (EF of ≥50%), diastolic dysfunction is assessed by a combinations as follows: E/E' greater than 14, E' on medial side of less than 7 cm/s or E' of less than 10 cm/ms, velocity of tricuspid regurgitation (TR) of more than 2.8 m/s, body surface area indexed left atrial volume of greater than 34 mL/m². In patients with a reduced EF (EF <50%), elevation of the left atrial pressure is assessed by combination of 3 parameters (E/E' >14, velocity of TR >2.8 m/s, indexed left atrial volume >34 mL/m²) when the transmitral flow pattern fulfills the criteria (a ratio of E to end-diastolic transmitral flow velocity [A] of >0.8 or <2; an E/A of ≤0.8 and E of >50 cm/s). Although these measures and classifications are recommended, they are still challenging in the clinical use because of limited data regarding diagnostic accuracy in emergent or urgent settings. Atrial fibrillation is the most frequent complication of AHF with a prevalence of 30% to 45%.[24] End-diastolic transmitral flow, which reflects atrial contraction, is abolished in patients with atrial fibrillation. The cycle length is variable, and left atrial size is enlarged regardless of LV filling pressure. Although dual gate Doppler imaging may overcome the heart rate variability for the assessment left atrial pressure elevation, the method is limited.[25] Therefore, stratification of diastolic dysfunction and left atrial pressure is limited and still challenging in patients with AHF with atrial fibrillation.

Elevation of Pulmonary Artery Hemodynamics

Causes of pulmonary hypertension is classified into 5 groups: pulmonary arterial hypertension (group 1), pulmonary hypertension owing to left heart disease (group 2), pulmonary hypertension owing to lung disease and/or hypoxia (group 3), chronic thromboembolic pulmonary hypertension and other pulmonary artery obstructions (group 4), and pulmonary hypertension with unclear and/or multifactorial mechanisms (group 5).[26] The most common types of pulmonary hypertension encountered in the ER setting are groups 2 and 4. Estimation of the pulmonary artery systolic pressure (PASP) using the simplified Bernoulli equation and an addition of right atrial pressure by respiratory distensibility of the IVC is the most common hemodynamic parameter in the diagnosis and

management of HF. In terms of severe TR, the simplified Bernoulli equation is not relevant to estimate PASP because of separation of tricuspid leaflet coaptation with laminar TR flow (**Fig. 5**). IVC diameter and respiratory distensibility is the most basic approach for the estimation of right atrial pressure and determination of intravascular volume status as a semiqualitative parameter. An IVC diameter of 2.1 cm or less with less than 50% collapse by sniffing suggests a right atrial pressure of 8 mm Hg (range, 5–10 mm Hg). An IVC diameter of 2.1 cm or less with 50% or greater collapse by sniffing suggests a right atrial pressure of 3 mm Hg (range, 0–5 mm Hg). An IVC diameter of greater than 2.1 cm with more than 50% collapse by sniffing suggests a right atrial pressure of 15 mm Hg (range, 10–20 mm Hg) (**Fig. 6**). The mean pulmonary artery pressure may be estimated as a summation of peak velocity of pulmonary regurgitation and estimated right atrial pressure.[27] The waveform of the pulse wave Doppler echocardiographic signal at the RV outflow tract is an indicative parameter for elevation of pulmonary vascular resistance. The double-peaked waveform is a qualitative sign of elevation pulmonary vascular resistance. The time to peak of pulse wave Doppler echocardiographic signal at RV outflow tract (acceleration time) and the ratio of acceleration time to RV ejection time are also classically useful quantitative parameters for elevation pulmonary vascular resistance and PASP.[28,29] Estimation of pulmonary vascular resistance can be determined a formula as follows[30]: pulmonary vascular resistance = (peak TR velocity/time – velocity interval of pulse wave Doppler echocardiographic signal at RV outflow tract) × 10 + 0.16.

The relationship between RV contraction by TAPSE and PASP (TAPSE/PASP ratio) as RV–PA coupling can reflect on the prognosis of patients with HF and pulmonary hypertension.[31,32]

FUTURE DIRECTIONS

Various studies have been published, but we still lack data regarding how to assess and manage patients with AHF particularly in the ER.[21] Novel technologies are expected to be more popular in emergency echocardiography. Devices are getting smaller. Knowledge must be organized and be comprehensive for diagnosis in the ER.

Two-dimensional strain imaging remains controversial regarding its clinical usefulness in emergency medicine.[33–36] Three-dimensional echocardiography may be a useful tool for emergency medicine. The images are showed from a pyramidal dataset avoiding through-plane effect.

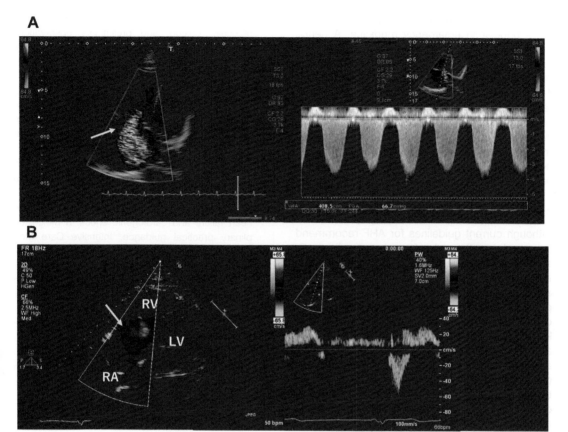

Fig. 5. RV-focused apical 4-chamber views showed 2 types of TR. (*A*) Color Doppler echocardiography showed moderate TR (*arrow*). Inset figure showed that continuous Doppler echocardiography presented elevated pressure gradient of TR with 66.7 mm Hg. (*B*) Color Doppler echocardiography showed severe TR with laminar flow (*arrow*). Inset figure showed that pulse wave Doppler echocardiography presented the TR flow. The laminar flow of TR is unsuitable for determination pressure gradient of TR by modified simplified Bernoulli equation. RA, right atrium.

However, the acquisition of images with the high temporal and spatial resolution is sometimes disturbed by observer skill and beat-to-beat variability. A deep learning method is a recent development in the technology associated with echocardiographic diagnosis. Further studies are required to achieve greater accuracy and better image quality and in various diseases, and various

Estimated RAP	3 mmHg (Normal: 0 – 5 mmHg)	8 mmHg (Intermediate: 5 – 10 mmHg)		15 mmHg (High: 10 – 20 mmHg)
IVC diameter	≤21 mm	≤21 mm	>21 mm	>21 mm
Collapse with sniff	≥50 %	<50 %	≥50 %	<50 %

Fig. 6. The right atrial pressure can be estimated by IVC diameter and distensibility. Composite figure presented 3° of estimated right atrial pressure by diameter of IVC and collapsibility with sniffing. RAP, right atrial pressure.

clinical settings for the new technique to become more popular in emergency medicine. A neural network approach provided high accuracy (96%) in the distinction of image views including partially obscured cardiac chambers from more than 14,000 echocardiographic images with wide-ranging subject background.[37] Recently, it has been reported that an automatic diagnosis of WMA by a deep convolutional neural network may be an adjunct tool in patients with ischemic heart disease, which is classified by 3 major coronary arteries.[38]

SUMMARY

Although current guidelines for AHF recommend using echocardiography for accurate diagnosis and subsequent immediate management of patients with AHF in the ER, little evidence for the applicability of patient selection has been reported. The observer should perform the echocardiographic study with a highly sophisticated knowledge of cardiovascular pathophysiology and plan an effective therapeutic strategy within a short time in the ER. The prevalence of HF is expected to increase in the advanced countries because of our aging society. Focused echocardiographic study and integration of conventional measures should be used more often in the diagnostic algorithm in the current emergent approach to AHF. In the future, advanced echocardiographic technologies (eg, strain imaging, 3-dimensional echocardiography) and automatic measurement (eg, LVEF, WMA) are expected to be used. Moreover, the neural network approach, which is based on massive echocardiographic information and medical knowledge, is very promising and its usefulness needs to be confirmed by further investigations focused on emergency medicine and patients' outcomes. It is concerning that artificial intelligence techniques may replace health care judgment by humans; however, it should be a supportive tool for every clinician including general practitioner as a novice clinical provider.

DISCLOSURE

The authors have nothing to disclose.

REFERENCES

1. Ambrosy AP, Fonarow GC, Butler J, et al. The global health and economic burden of hospitalizations for heart failure: lessons learned from hospitalized heart failure registries. J Am Coll Cardiol 2014;63(12): 1123–33.
2. Adams KF Jr, Fonarow GC, Emerman CL, et al. Characteristics and outcomes of patients hospitalized for heart failure in the United States: rationale, design, and preliminary observations from the first 100,000 cases in the Acute Decompensated Heart Failure National Registry (ADHERE). Am Heart J 2005;149(2):209–16.
3. Ponikowski P, Voors AA, Anker SD, et al. 2016 ESC guidelines for the diagnosis and treatment of acute and chronic heart failure: the task force for the diagnosis and treatment of acute and chronic heart failure of the European Society of Cardiology (ESC) Developed with the special contribution of the Heart Failure Association (HFA) of the ESC. Eur Heart J 2016;37(27):2129–200.
4. Mebazaa A, Tolppanen H, Mueller C, et al. Acute heart failure and cardiogenic shock: a multidisciplinary practical guidance. Intensive Care Med 2016;42(2):147–63.
5. Neskovic AN, Hagendorff A, Lancellotti P, et al. Emergency echocardiography: the European Association of Cardiovascular Imaging recommendations. Eur Heart J Cardiovasc Imaging 2013;14(1):1–11.
6. Permanyer-Miralda G. Acute pericardial disease: approach to the aetiologic diagnosis. Heart 2004; 90(3):252–4.
7. Woodring JH. Distribution of pleural effusion in congestive heart failure: what is atypical? South Med J 2005;98(5):518–23.
8. Pivetta E, Goffi A, Lupia E, et al. Lung ultrasound-implemented diagnosis of acute decompensated heart failure in the ED: a SIMEU multicenter study. Chest 2015;148(1):202–10.
9. Lichtenstein D, Meziere G. A lung ultrasound sign allowing bedside distinction between pulmonary edema and COPD: the comet-tail artifact. Intensive Care Med 1998;24(12):1331–4.
10. Volpicelli G, Cardinale L, Garofalo G, et al. Usefulness of lung ultrasound in the bedside distinction between pulmonary edema and exacerbation of COPD. Emerg Radiol 2008;15(3):145–51.
11. Volpicelli G, Elbarbary M, Blaivas M, et al. International evidence-based recommendations for point-of-care lung ultrasound. Intensive Care Med 2012; 38(4):577–91.
12. Cikes M, Solomon SD. Beyond ejection fraction: an integrative approach for assessment of cardiac structure and function in heart failure. Eur Heart J 2016;37(21):1642–50.
13. Paczynska M, Sobieraj P, Burzynski L, et al. Tricuspid annulus plane systolic excursion (TAPSE) has superior predictive value compared to right ventricular to left ventricular ratio in normotensive patients with acute pulmonary embolism. Arch Med Sci 2016;12(5):1008–14.
14. Frea S, Pidello S, Bovolo V, et al. Prognostic incremental role of right ventricular function in acute decompensation of advanced chronic heart failure. Eur J Heart Fail 2016;18(5):564–72.

15. Bodez D, Ternacle J, Guellich A, et al. Prognostic value of right ventricular systolic function in cardiac amyloidosis. Amyloid 2016;23(3):158–67.

16. Kjaergaard J, Iversen KK, Akkan D, et al. Predictors of right ventricular function as measured by tricuspid annular plane systolic excursion in heart failure. Cardiovasc Ultrasound 2009;7:51.

17. Forfia PR, Fisher MR, Mathai SC, et al. Tricuspid annular displacement predicts survival in pulmonary hypertension. Am J Respir Crit Care Med 2006; 174(9):1034–41.

18. Lang RM, Badano LP, Mor-Avi V, et al. Recommendations for cardiac chamber quantification by echocardiography in adults: an update from the American Society of Echocardiography and the European Association of Cardiovascular Imaging. J Am Soc Echocardiogr 2015;28(1):1–39.e14.

19. Skyba DM, Camarano G, Goodman NC, et al. Hemodynamic characteristics, myocardial kinetics and microvascular rheology of FS-069, a second-generation echocardiographic contrast agent capable of producing myocardial opacification from a venous injection. J Am Coll Cardiol 1996; 28(5):1292–300.

20. Zehender M, Kasper W, Kauder E, et al. Right ventricular infarction as an independent predictor of prognosis after acute inferior myocardial infarction. N Engl J Med 1993;328(14):981–8.

21. Ferre RM, Chioncel O, Pang PS, et al. Acute heart failure: the role of focused emergency cardiopulmonary ultrasound in identification and early management. Eur J Heart Fail 2015;17(12):1223–7.

22. Nagueh SF, Middleton KJ, Kopelen HA, et al. Doppler tissue imaging: a noninvasive technique for evaluation of left ventricular relaxation and estimation of filling pressures. J Am Coll Cardiol 1997; 30(6):1527–33.

23. Nagueh SF, Smiseth OA, Appleton CP, et al. Recommendations for the evaluation of left ventricular diastolic function by echocardiography: an update from the American Society of Echocardiography and the European Association of Cardiovascular Imaging. J Am Soc Echocardiogr 2016;29(4):277–314.

24. Abualnaja S, Podder M, Hernandez AF, et al. Acute heart failure and atrial fibrillation: insights from the acute study of clinical effectiveness of nesiritide in decompensated heart failure (ASCEND-HF) trial. J Am Heart Assoc 2015;4(8):e002092.

25. Kusunose K, Yamada H, Nishio S, et al. Clinical utility of single-beat E/e' obtained by simultaneous recording of flow and tissue Doppler velocities in atrial fibrillation with preserved systolic function. JACC Cardiovasc Imaging 2009;2(10):1147–56.

26. Simonneau G, Montani D, Celermajer DS, et al. Haemodynamic definitions and updated clinical classification of pulmonary hypertension. Eur Respir J 2019;53(1) [pii:1801913].

27. Masuyama T, Kodama K, Kitabatake A, et al. Continuous-wave doppler echocardiographic detection of pulmonary regurgitation and its application to noninvasive estimation of pulmonary artery pressure. Circulation 1986;74(3):484–92.

28. Kitabatake A, Inoue M, Asao M, et al. Noninvasive evaluation of pulmonary hypertension by a pulsed doppler technique. Circulation 1983;68(2): 302–9.

29. Yared K, Noseworthy P, Weyman AE, et al. Pulmonary artery acceleration time provides an accurate estimate of systolic pulmonary arterial pressure during transthoracic echocardiography. J Am Soc Echocardiogr 2011;24(6):687–92.

30. Abbas AE, Fortuin FD, Schiller NB, et al. A simple method for noninvasive estimation of pulmonary vascular resistance. J Am Coll Cardiol 2003;41(6): 1021–7.

31. Tello K, Axmann J, Ghofrani HA, et al. Relevance of the TAPSE/PASP ratio in pulmonary arterial hypertension. Int J Cardiol 2018;266:229–35.

32. Guazzi M, Bandera F, Pelissero G, et al. Tricuspid annular plane systolic excursion and pulmonary arterial systolic pressure relationship in heart failure: an index of right ventricular contractile function and prognosis. Am J Physiol Heart Circ Physiol 2013; 305(9):H1373–81.

33. Reardon L, Scheels WJ, Singer AJ, et al. Feasibility and accuracy of speckle tracking echocardiography in emergency department patients. Am J Emerg Med 2018;36(12):2254–9.

34. Shiran A, Blondheim DS, Shimoni S, et al. Two-dimensional strain echocardiography for diagnosing chest pain in the emergency room: a multicentre prospective study by the Israeli echo research group. Eur Heart J Cardiovasc Imaging 2017; 18(9):1016–24.

35. Favot M, Courage C, Ehrman R, et al. Strain echocardiography in acute cardiovascular diseases. West J Emerg Med 2016;17(1):54–60.

36. Bagger T, Sloth E, Jakobsen CJ. Left ventricular longitudinal function assessed by speckle tracking ultrasound from a single apical imaging plane. Crit Care Res Pract 2012;2012:361824.

37. Zhang J, Gajjala S, Agrawal P, et al. Fully automated echocardiogram interpretation in clinical practice. Circulation 2018;138(16):1623–35.

38. Kusunose K, Abe T, Haga A, et al. A deep learning approach for assessment of regional wall motion abnormality from echocardiographic images. JACC Cardiovasc Imaging 2019. https://doi.org/10.1016/j.jcmg.2019.02.024 [pii:S1936-878X(19) 30318-3].

How to Bail Out Patients with Severe Acute Myocardial Infarction

Yuichiro Toma, MD

KEYWORDS

- Cardiogenic shock • Acute myocardial infarction • Mechanical circulatory support

KEY POINTS

- Early diagnosis and early revascularization are important for favorable outcome in patients with acute myocardial infarction (AMI) plus cardiogenic shock.
- In patients with severe AMI, it is critically important to elucidate and stabilize hemodynamics for end-organ perfusion and its protection with appropriate therapeutic actions.
- Medical therapy and mechanical circulatory supports should be used with an understanding of their properties, indications, contraindications, adverse effects, and limitations.

INTRODUCTION

Acute myocardial infarction (AMI) was previously a dangerous clinical event with high mortality. The development of primary percutaneous coronary intervention (PCI) has dramatically improved mortality rates from the 1980s to the present.[1,2] However, until now, the rate of coexisting cardiogenic shock (CS) in AMI has been reported to be 5% to 8%.[3] Patients with CS have severe coronary artery disease. It was reported that 53% these patients had triple vessels disease, and 16% them had left main trunk (LMT) disease.[4] The mortality rate of CS caused by AMI is decreasing year by year; however, it is still about 50%, and the prognosis of the patients is still poor.[5] The prognosis can be improved by appropriate drug therapy and mechanical circulatory support (MCS) for such serious conditions following AMI. This article describes the management of such patients.

DEFINITION

The criteria of Myocardial Infarction Research Units of the National Heart and Lung Institute (MIRU) define CS as hypotension (a systolic blood pressure of <90 mm Hg for at least 30 minutes or the need for supportive measures to maintain a systolic blood pressure of ≥90 mm Hg) and end-organ hypoperfusion (cool extremities or a urine output of <20 mL per hour, and disturbance of consciousness).[6] The hemodynamic criteria (Forrester classification) are defined as a cardiac index of no more than 2.2 L/min/m² of body-surface area and a pulmonary-capillary wedge pressure of 18 mm Hg or higher.[7] In particular, large anterior myocardial infarction is likely to fall into cardiogenic shock. Creatine kinase (CK), troponin T (TnT), troponin I (TnI), and creatine kinase MB (CK-MB) are known to be correlated with myocardial infarction size.[8,9] Both CK and CK-MB are important biomarkers representing the severity and mortality of AMI.

Etiology

Identification of the cause of CS during diagnosis is necessary in order to provide appropriate treatment. Cardiogenic shock in AMI has several causes. **Box 1** shows the known causes of AMI.[3] The factor of coronary artery in **Box 1** damages the myocardium directory. Acute extensive

Funding Sources: None.
Department of Cardiovascular Medicine, Nephrology, and Neurology, Faculty of Medicine, University of the Ryukyus, 207 Uehara, Nishihara-cho, Okinawa 903-0215, Japan
E-mail address: asikaga@yahoo.co.jp

Box 1
Causes of cardiogenic shock following acute myocardial infarction

Causes of cardiogenic shock with AMI

Directly impairing cardiac contractile function by acute coronary ischemia

Dynamic LV outflow tract obstruction

Acute dysrhythmia secondary to acute ischemia

Acute ventricular septal perforation

Acute mitral regurgitation caused by mitral valve papillary muscle rupture/ischemia.

LV free wall rupture

Pericardial tamponade

Type A dissection involving coronary arteries

Right ventricle infarction

anterior infarction with the left main trunk (LMT) involvement and a proximal lesion in the left anterior descending artery (LAD) can contribute to shock because of widespread myocardial damage. Coronary revascularization is the best treatment for left ventricle failure, left ventricular outflow tract obstruction (LVOT), and lethal arrhythmia caused by ischemia. The culprit of AMI at the distal branch of LAD might cause LVOT obstruction, because the septal wall motion may change hyperkinetic like Takotsubo cardiomyopathy. Although that change may lead to CS owing to reduced stroke volume, revascularization with PCI will be able to improve the left ventricle wall motion of apical ballooning site, which will release LVOT obstruction, eventually. Symptomatic treatment is the only option if cardiogenic shock is not improved by revascularization. In the SHOCK Trial Registry, the rate of LV failure was 78.5%; the rate of isolated right heart failure was 6.9%, and mechanical complication caused by acute mitral regurgitation due to papillary muscle rupture was 6.9%. The ventricular septal perforation (VSP) rate was 3.9%, and cardiac tamponade or LV perforation was 1.4%.[10] In general, CS often occurs when the infarction size of the left ventricle is more than 40%. Although the cut-off values of CK-MB and TnT for future CS have been unknown, previous reports indicated that CK-MB greater than 800 U/L and TnT greater than 15 mcg/L may lead to high-probability of cardiogenic shock after AMI.[8,9] However, the peak values of CK-MB and TnT occur 24 to 72 hours after the onset of AMI, so the timing of its measurements should be considered.

FROM INITIAL DIAGNOSIS TO CORONARY REVASCULARIZATION

Early revascularization is known to improve the prognosis in AMI patients.[11] A prognosis comparison between an early revascularization enforcement group (PCI or coronary artery bypass grafting [CABG]) and nonenforcement group (conservative treatment) was performed in AMI patients who had cardiogenic shock caused by LV dysfunction in the SHOCK Trial registry.[12] The 6-month mortality rate was significantly lower in early revascularization group. If AMI is suspected, a brief and accurate medical history should be obtained from the first medical contact immediately after AMI. After arrival at the hospital, it is necessary to record electrocardiogram and echocardiogram promptly and to perform thrombolysis and revascularization.

Percutaneous Coronary Intervention

Historically, thrombolytic therapy has been the mainstream of treatment for AMI, but it was reported that primary PCI had better prognosis than thrombolytic therapy.[11] In the guidelines on ST elevation myocardial infarction (STEMI) of the American Heart Association (AHA), Primary PCI is recommended for AMI including CS. The class I recommendation of the ESC/EACTS on reperfusion strategy of STEMI is to perform early revascularization by primary PCI.[13,14] The prognosis of AMI with shock was improved when the time to primary PCI was shorter.[15] It is important to shorten total ischemic time from the onset to reperfusion in STEMI including shock state. When door-to-balloon time was less than 90 minutes in the patients who presented in a hospital within 2 hours from the onset, the prognosis was significantly better.[16] For best results, the door-to-balloon time should be less than 90 minutes for primary PCI.

Coronary Artery Bypass Grafting

Another method available for revascularization is coronary artery bypass grafting (CABG). Recently, as a method of coronary revascularization, a report has shown that there was no significant difference in prognosis between PCI and CABG for unprotected LMT and multivessel disease.[17] CABG should be considered to provide a better prognosis than PCI, in patients with diabetic mellitus, complex lesions with other multivessel lesions, and LMT.[18] However, in AMI with CS, CABG is performed in few situations, because PCI can be performed in many cases in a shorter time compared with CABG. When mechanical surgical repair is required in cases such as VSP, acute mitral valve reflux caused by papillary muscle rupture and left ventricle free wall rupture, CABG should be considered at the same time.[19]

MEDICAL THERAPY FOR CARDIOGENIC SHOCK

At present, little is known about cardiogenic shock associated with severe AMI. When MCS or PCI is performed, medical therapy is used concurrently in all cases. For CS, medical therapy is always necessary. **Fig. 1** shows the 2016 ESC heart failure guidelines[20] recommended for cardiogenic shock. When AMI develops CS, at first it should be confirmed if the patient is hypervolemic. Rapid fluid replacement is performed with saline and lactated Ringer solution without reaching a state of hypervolemia. The patient should subsequently be given inotropes if the state of shock continues. Conventionally, catecholamines have been used as main inotropes. Noradrenaline, dopamine (precursor of noradrenaline), and dobutamine have β1 stimulating effects, but in particular, noradrenaline also has strong α1 and strong vasopressor activity. In addition, noradrenaline is less likely to raise heart rate compared with dopamine. A randomized controlled trial, SOAP-II, compared noradrenaline with dopamine for treatment of CS[21] in first-line treatment of patients of CS. The mortality rate at day 28 was the primary endpoint and was not significantly different between the 2 groups. However, incidence of adverse events associated with arrhythmia was significantly higher in the dopamine group. At present,

administration of noradrenaline is recommended for hypotension in the 2016 ESC heart failure guidelines. The 2013 ACCF/AHA guidelines noted that dopamine might be associated with an adverse event.[22] Indications of inotropes should be considered when the previously mentioned MIRU criteria will be matched, or when the lactic acid level is elevated (>2.0 mmol/L)[23] as an evidence of poor perfusion of other end organs. The purpose of administering the inotropes is to support perfusion of major end organs. In order to obtain the beneficial effect of inotropes, it may be not only to measure cardiac output with a Swan-Ganz catheter but also to evaluate clinical symptoms and/or laboratory data related to hypoperfusion in end organs, such as physical examinations for peripheral perfusion, renal function, liver function, lactate level, and mixed venous oxygen saturation. Without severe infection or anemia, SvO_2 and $ScvO_2$ are also good clinical indicators of perfusion of end-organs.[24]

However, the effects of the inotropes have still remained controversial. It has been reported that inotropes were able to improve hemodynamics and clinical symptoms because of increase LV contractility in patients with CS plus progressing end organ damage.[25] Despite its beneficial effects on myocardial contractility, the adverse effects of inotropic therapy, such as arrhythmias or increased myocardial oxygen consumption, may be associated with increased mortality.[26] For example, some clinical studies have demonstrated that dobutamine and/or PDE-III inhibitor did not improve long-term prognosis in patients with acute decompensated heart failure or AMI, unexpectedly.[27,28] In general, increased myocardial oxygen consumption by inotropes may lead to fatal arrhythmias and/or ischemic events in patients with AMI. Therefore, inotropes should be completed in lower-dose and in a short time, appropriately. The clinical dose of dobutamine is usually around 2.0 μg/kg/min, because dobutamine greater than 5.0 μg/kg/min may be able to increase atrial fibrillation and ventricular tachyarrhythmias.[29] Levosimendan, a PDE-III inhibitor, might be able to improve hemodynamics without adverse events in AMI patients who have already taken β-blockers[30] It has been reported that hemodynamics and prognosis were improved by the combination treatment with PDE-III inhibitors and dobutamine.[31] If the treatment with inotropes might be prolonged, the transition to MCS should be considered an appropriate phase. In patients with severe AMI, it is critically important to elucidate and stabilize hemodynamics for the end organ perfusion and its protection with appropriate therapeutic actions.

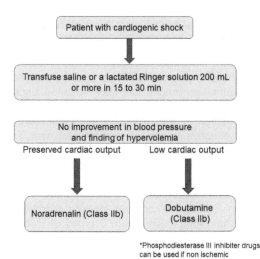

Fig. 1. Algorithm for medical therapy management of cardiogenic shock.

INTRA-AORTIC BALLOON PUMPING

Conventionally, intra-aortic balloon pumping (IABP) has been often used as a mechanical circulatory support for maintaining hemodynamics in patients with CS. IABP has 2 effects: systolic unloading and diastolic augmentation for supporting cardiac function. In the systolic phase, the balloon is rapidly deflated to reduce the afterload. This effect contributes to a decrease in LV work load and a decrease in LV myocardial oxygen demand. In the diastolic phase, the balloon placed in the descending aorta is expanded to increase the central aortic pressure, resulting in increased coronary perfusion pressure and blood flow.[32] This effect is enhanced when the microvascular circulatory reserve is greatly reduced, such as in CS and prolonged hypotension.[33] The supporting circulatory volume is about 15% to 20% (0.5–1 L/min) of the whole-body effective plasma volume. The advantages of IABP are that it is only minimally invasive, can be inserted in a short time, is not very difficult to manage, and has few complications at the insertion site. Previously, IABP was employed for CS when thrombolytic therapy was widely used. Subsequent observational studies reported the usefulness of IABP for AMI patients with CS.[34] In various guidelines, IABP was recommended as a class I measure. However, with time, primary PCI became mainstream and continues to be used at the present. It is important to revisit the role of IABP. The IABP-SHOCK II trial was a randomized controlled trial using IABP either before the PCI or immediately after the PCI in AMI.[35] This study randomly assigned AMI patients with CS to 2 groups; 1 group received IABP and the other group (non-IABP) I. The study compared the prognosis after revascularization. As a result, the 30-day mortality rate was 39.7% in the IABP group and 41.3% in the non-IABP group (P=.69). The 12-month mortality rate was 52.0% in the IABP group and 51.0% in the non-IABP group (P=.91). As a result of this study, use of IABP in AMI with CS decreased. The recommendations were changed to class IIa for CS with unstable hemodynamics caused by mechanical complications, and routine use for CS changed to class III measure.[36] A subanalysis of the CRISP-AMI study suggested that there was a significant improvement in the 6-month mortality rate in patients with persistent myocardial ischemia or large infarctions.[37] However, following the development of percutaneous LV assist device (LVAD) such as Impella and Tandem Heart and down-grading in the guidelines, the usage rate of IABP was reduced to less than 30%[38] in the United States and less than 25%[39] in the United Kingdom.

MECHANICAL CIRCULATORY SUPPORT

MCS is required if medical therapy cannot maintain appropriate hemodynamics in CS. However, even if short-term MCS was used and then cardiac function was not recovered, mid- to long-term MCS must also be considered. Short-term use devices include IABP, venoarterial extracorporeal membrane oxygenation (VA-ECMO), percutaneous LVAD (pLVAD) (Impella Abiomed, Danvers, USA, and Tandem Heart Cardiac Assist, USA). In addition to AMI, these short-term MCS devices are used in acute myocarditis, acute exacerbation of chronic heart failure, low cardiac output after cardiovascular surgery, and fatal sustained arrhythmias. It is important to know when to use these short-term MCS devices. The standard criteria for use of MCS is not clear, because the clinical state of CS patients changes frequently. Primary PCI is usually preferred, but if the patient is in CS, MCS insertion should be considered to stabilize hemodynamics over PCI. Hemodynamic failure leads to unfortunate outcomes such as hypoxic encephalopathy. Previously, IABP and VA-ECMO were the main options. Currently, the available options for transcutaneous MCS are pLVAD such as Impella and Tandem Heart and right ventricle assist devices such as Impella RP and Tandem Heart RVAD, and these are being used more frequently. The algorithm for cardiac support with CS is shown in **Fig. 2**. Each MCS modality has its own advantages. There are left heart assistance, right heart assistance, and oxygenation assistance devices, and each has to be used properly according to the clinical condition (**Fig. 3**).

Extracorporeal Membrane Oxygenation

Research on extracorporeal membrane oxygenation (ECMO) began in the 1970s.[40] Initially, oxygenation was the main purpose, and patients with acute respiratory failure were indicated. Especially for neonatal medicine, ECMO has achieved good results[41] and ECMO is presently established as an effective treatment method. However, for adults with acute respiratory failure, the results are poor[42] and therefore, it is not a commonly used treatment. On the other hand, the use of ECMO for extracorporeal cardiopulmonary resuscitation (ECPR) has become popular worldwide since the 1980s.[43] There are 2 types of ECMO: VA-ECMO (venous removal-aorta transmission) and VV-ECMO (venous removal-venous transmission). VA-ECMO is used to support circulation. VA-ECMO removes venous blood from the right

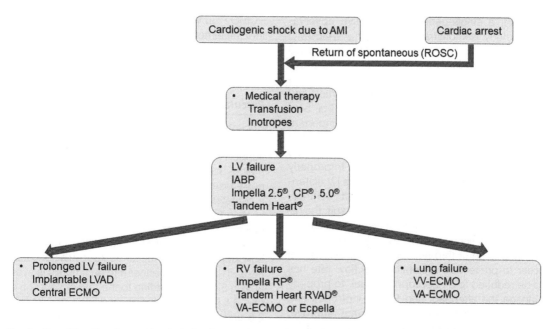

Fig. 2. Algorithm for the mechanical circulatory support devices for AMI with cardiogenic shock.

atrium, oxygenates it, and pumps it back to the descending aorta. VA-ECMO removes venous blood from the right atrium and pumps oxygenated blood retrogradely into the femoral artery. In AMI, VA-ECMO is indicated for patients who still cannot recover from shock using IABP, or who have cardiac arrest, or VT/VF storm that cannot maintain hemodynamics. Circulatory failure caused by mechanical complications in AMI is also considered an indication. VSP may result in decreased forward ejection cardiac output and circulatory failure even though oxygenation is maintained because of shunted blood flow from the left ventricle to the right ventricle. VA-ECMO is effective, because blood can be removed from

the right atrium, where there is volume overload.[44] As a guideline, VA-ECMO should be used for about 1 to 7 days, as there is a high possibility of complications with long-term use. If cardiac function does not recover after VA-ECMO insertion, consider cardiac transplantation, implantable LVAD, or central VA-ECMO.[45] A prospective observational study was conducted to investigate the effectiveness of ECMO in patients with out-of-hospital cardiac arrest caused by AMI or arrhythmia. The study suggested that VA-ECMO was an effective procedure.[46] In the study, 11.2% of patients in the ECMO group returned to social life 6 months after cardiac arrest, compared with 2.6% of patients in the non-ECMO group. In

LV failure   **RV failure**

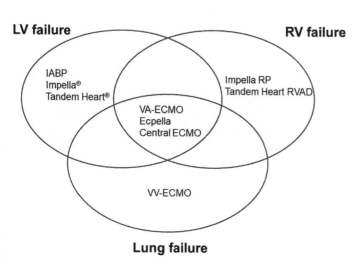

Fig. 3. Selecting a short-term supportive device according to the clinical scenario.

addition, a single-center retrospective observational study demonstrated that using VA-ECMO in ACS patients was not effective for severe CS but was effective for moderate shock.[47] The prognostic factors of ACS patients relating to VA-ECMO were the time to VA-ECMO insertion and whether reperfusion was successful.[48] For best outcome for AMI patients with CS, it is important not to hesitate to insert VA-ECMO and to perform coronary revascularization earlier. There are several problems with VA-ECMO. Improperly increasing the flow of VA-ECMO causes LV distention, leading to an increase in left ventricle end-diastolic pressure (LVEDP). As a result, the recovery of the left ventricle is delayed, LV distention causes complications such as pulmonary edema and formation of thrombus in the left ventricle. In order to prevent LV distention, the flow rate has to be reduced to an appropriate level, to properly manage the afterload, and to use inotropes and IABP. If LV distention still does not improve, consider Impella insertion, insertion into LV or LA vent under thoracotomy, or transition to LVAD. VA-ECMO also has frequent bleeding complications. Use of anticoagulant therapy during VA-ECMO is indispensable to prevent in-circuit thrombosis and systemic embolism, and coagulation factors were depleted by activation of the coagulation cascade and ECMO circuit. Hemorrhagic complications during VA-ECMO procedure can be fatal.[49] Other complications such as lower limb ischemia are frequent and require attention. It has been reported that lower limb ischemia appeared in 70% of patients who received VA-ECMO.[50] In VA-ECMO, a thick catheter is inserted into the femoral artery compared with that in IABP, which may be fatal because of myonephrotic metabolic syndrome (MNMS) associated with lower limb ischemia.

Percutaneous Left Ventricular Assist Devices

Recently, percutaneous LVADs (pLVADs) have been used as a standard mechanical circulatory support for CS. Impella and Tandem Heart are mainly used for pLVAD. Impella is a percutaneously insertable heart failure treatment device on a catheter mounted with a small axial pump. The suction hole located in the left ventricle sucks up blood using a small axial flow pump implanted in the pigtail catheter and ejects it from the outflow hole located beyond the aortic valve in a nonpulsatile and antegrade manner (**Fig. 4**). Impella is available in 3 types according to the rate of flow, 2.5 L/min, 3.5 L/min (Impella CP), and 5.0 L/min. Impella 2.5 and Impella CP can be inserted through the femoral artery with puncture. However, Impella 5.0 must be inserted through the subclavian artery with cut-down by surgeons. The supporting flow rate of various mechanical supportive devices including Impella is shown in **Fig. 5**. Impella can monitor blood pressure using pressure waveforms. Impella has 3 circulatory assist effects following: unloading LV pressure and volume, reduction in LV wall stress, and decrease in myocardial oxygen consumption. Impella partially supports the cardiac output unlike treatment with inotropes or IABP. The mechanism is considered to decrease myocardial oxygen consumption by

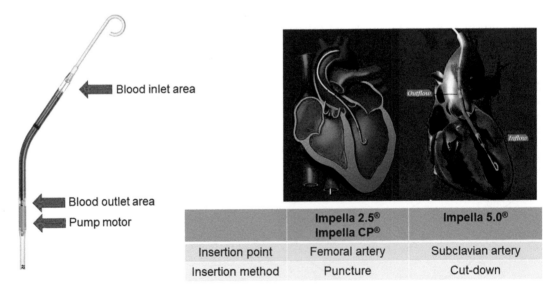

	Impella 2.5® Impella CP®	Impella 5.0®
Insertion point	Femoral artery	Subclavian artery
Insertion method	Puncture	Cut-down

Fig. 4. Percutaneous left ventricular assist device. Impella 2.5 inserted from femoral artery, whereas Impella 5.0 inserted from subclavian artery. (*Product images courtesy of* Abiomed Japan K.K., Tokyo, Japan.)

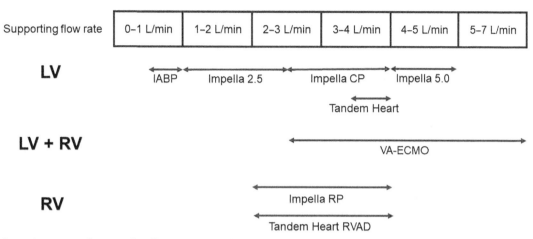

Supporting flow rate	0–1 L/min	1–2 L/min	2–3 L/min	3–4 L/min	4–5 L/min	5–7 L/min

LV

IABP   Impella 2.5   Impella CP   Impella 5.0

Tandem Heart

LV + RV

VA-ECMO

RV

Impella RP

Tandem Heart RVAD

Fig. 5. Summary of supporting flow rate in mechanical circulatory supportive devices.

reducing the potential energy and external work indicated by the PV-loop area while maintaining systemic circulation.[51] In a porcine myocardial infarction model, Impella reduced the infarct size by reducing myocardial oxygen consumption in addition to improving coronary blood flow.[52] In a clinical study, high-risk PCI patients were randomly divided into 2 groups; 1 group was treated with IABP and another group with Impella 2.5.[53] There was a trend toward decreased major adverse events, but was not statistically significant after 30 days; however, after 90 days of follow-up, there was a strong tend toward lower incidence of major adverse events in the Impella group compared with the group receiving IABP. These data support the safety and utility of Impella in AMI patients. In the USpella trial, the hemodynamics of the patients with CS who did not improve with inotropes and IABP after AMI was significantly improved when Impella 2.5 was used.[54] In the MACH II trial, patients with acute anterior wall STEMI in the group using Impella 2.5 had significantly improved cardiac function compared with standard of care treatment.[55] Impella 5.0 was reported to be safe and effective in treatment of CS after cardiopulmonary-assisted circulation withdrawal in the RECOVER I trial.[56] There are 2 studies that directly compared IABP and Impella. The ISAR-SHOCK trial[57] performed in Germany enrolled AMI patients with CS. Patients were randomized into 2 groups, IABP and Impella 2.5. The change in cardiac index was compared 30 minutes after the start of circulation assist. The IMPRESS severe shock trial[58] was performed at 2 sites in the Netherlands and Norway. AMI patients with CS, including cardiac arrest, were randomly divided into 2 groups, IABP and Impella CP. The patient groups were compared at 30 days and at 6 months for mortality; there was no significant difference between the 2 groups. In order to maximize the effects of Impella, it is desirable to start Impella relatively early.[59] However, if the patient has severe respiratory failure, Impella alone is not sufficient, and VA-ECMO is necessary to keep proper oxygenation. This combination is called Ecpella, and it reduces LV afterload and pulmonary congestion with oxygenation support.[60,61] Because Ecpella can also provide flow assistance for VA-ECMO, Impella 5.0 is not always necessary, and Impella 2.5 or Impella CP is sufficient. Impella is a useful device; however, its position in the left ventricle may change, and the flow rate may be insufficient. In addition, because Impella has a risk for hemolytic anemia and thrombosis, it should be carefully managed. Tamdem Heart is a device with almost the same mechanism. There is no large trial with Tandem Heart. In a small study as with Impella, the cardiac index improved compared with IABP, but the mortality rate was not significantly improved.[62]

SUMMARY

The treatment of severe AMI has changed over time. The new mechanical circulatory assist devices such as Impella and Tandem Heart have appeared, and the options for treatment are expanding. Early revascularization is a priority for severe AMI, but there is no clear standard on how to use these new devices and existing therapies for severe AMI with CS. When treating AMI patients with CS, one should select treatment methods considering tissue perfusion, organ protection, oxygenation, myocardial protection, and right heart function.

DISCLOSURE

The author has nothing to disclose.

REFERENCES

1. Dégano IR, Salomaa V, Veronesi G, et al, Acute Myocardial Infarction Trends in Europe (AMITIE) Study Investigators. Twenty-five-year trends in myocardial infarction attack and mortality rates, and case-fatality, in six European populations. Heart 2015;101:1413–21.

2. Schmidt M, Jacobsen JB, Lash TL, et al. 25 year trends in first time hospitalisation for acute myocardial infarction, subsequent short and long term mortality, and the prognostic impact of sex and comorbidity: a Danish nationwide cohort study. BMJ 2012;344:e356.

3. Tharmaratnam D, Nolan J, Jain A. Management of cardiogenic shock complicating acute coronary syndromes. Heart 2013;99:1614–23.

4. Wong SC, Sanborn T, Sleeper LA, et al. Angiographic findings and clinical correlates in patients with cardiogenic shock complicating acute myocardial infarction: a report from the SHOCK Trial Registry. SHould we emergently revascularize Occluded Coronaries for cardiogenic shocK? J Am Coll Cardiol 2000;36:1077–83.

5. Werdan K, Gielen S, Ebelt H, et al. Mechanical circulatory support in cardiogenic shock. Eur Heart J 2014;35:156–67.

6. Swan HJ, Forrester JS, Diamond G, et al. Hemodynamic spectrum of myocardial infarction and cardiogenic shock. A conceptual model. Circulation 1972;45:1097–110.

7. Forrester JS, Diamond G, Chatterjee K, et al. Medical therapy of acute myocardial infarction by application of hemodynamic subsets (second of two parts). N Engl J Med 1976;295(25):1404–13.

8. Dohi T, Maehara A, Brener SJ. Utility of peak creatine kinase-MB measurements in predicting myocardial infarct size, left ventricular dysfunction, and outcome after first anterior wall acute myocardial infarction (from the INFUSE-AMI trial). Am J Cardiol 2015;115(5):563–70.

9. Byrne RA, Ndrepepa G, Braun S, et al. Peak cardiac troponin-T level, scintigraphic myocardial infarct size and one-year prognosis in patients undergoing primary percutaneous coronary intervention for acute myocardial infarction. Am J Cardiol 2010;106(9):1212–7.

10. Hochman JS, Buller CE, Sleeper LA, et al. Cardiogenic shock complicating acute myocardial infarction–etiologies, management and outcome: a report from the SHOCK Trial Registry. SHould we emergently revascularize Occluded Coronaries for cardiogenic shocK? J Am Coll Cardiol 2000;36:1063–70.

11. Keeley EC, Boura JA, Grines CL. Primary angioplasty versus intravenous thrombolytic therapy for acute myocardial infarction: a quantitative review of 23 randomized trials. Lancet 2003;361:13–20.

12. Hochman JS, Sleeper LA, Webb JG, et al. Early revascularization in acute myocardial infarction complicated by cardiogenic shock. SHOCK Investigators. SHould we emergently revascularize occluded coronaries for cardiogenic shocK. N Engl J Med 1999;341:625–34.

13. Neumann FJ, Sousa-Uva M, Ahlsson A, et al. 2018 ESC/EACTS Guidelines on myocardial revascularization. Eur Heart J 2019;40:87–165.

14. O'Gara PT, Kushner FG, Ascheim DD, et al. 2013 ACCF/AHA guideline for the management of ST-elevation myocardial infarction. A report of the American College of Cardiology Foundation/American Heart Association Task Force on Practice Guidelines. J Am Coll Cardiol 2013;61(4):e78–140.

15. Scholz KH, Maier SKG, Maier LS, et al. Impact of treatment delay on mortality in ST-segment elevation myocardial infarction (STEMI) patients presenting with and without hemodynamic instability: results from the German prospective, multicenter FITT-STEMI trial. Eur Heart J 2018;39:1065–74.

16. Shiomi H, Nakagawa Y, Morimoto T, et al, CREDO-Kyoto AMI investigators. Association of onset to balloon and door to balloon time with long term clinical outcome in patients with ST elevation acute myocardial infarction having primary percutaneous coronary intervention: observational study. BMJ 2012;344:e3257.

17. Mohr FW, Morice MC, Kappetein AP, et al. Coronary artery bypass graft surgery versus percutaneous coronary intervention in patients with three-vessel disease and left main coronary disease: 5-year follow-up of the randomised, clinical SYNTAX trial. Lancet 2013;381(9867):629–38.

18. Head SJ, Milojevic M, Daemen J, et al. Mortality after coronary artery bypass grafting versus percutaneous coronary intervention with stenting for coronary artery disease: a pooled analysis of individual patient data. Lancet 2018;391:939–48.

19. Thompson CR, Buller CE, Sleeper LA, et al. Cardiogenic shock due to acute severe mitral regurgitation complicating acute myocardial infarction: a report from the SHOCK Trial Registry. SHould we use emergently revascularize Occluded Coronaries in cardiogenic shocK? J Am Coll Cardiol 2000;36:1104–9.

20. Ponikowski P, Voors AA, Anker SD, et al. 2016 ESC Guidelines for the diagnosis and treatment of acute and chronic heart failure: the Task Force for the diagnosis and treatment of acute and chronic heart failure of the European Society of Cardiology (ESC) Developed with the special contribution of the Heart Failure Association (HFA) of the ESC. Eur Heart J 2016;37:2129–200.

21. De Backer D, Biston P, Devriendt J, et al. Comparison of dopamine and norepinephrine in the treatment of shock. N Engl J Med 2010;362:779–89.

22. O'Gara PT, Kushner FG, Ascheim DD, et al. 2013 ACCF/AHA guideline for the management of ST-elevation myocardial infarction: a report of the American College of Cardiology Foundation/American Heart Association Task Force on Practice Guidelines. Circulation 2013;127:e362–425.

23. Khosravani H, Shahpori R, Stelfox HT, et al. Occurrence and adverse effect on outcome of hyperlactatemia in the critically ill. Crit Care 2009; 13(3):R90.

24. Cournand A, Riley RL, Breed ES, et al. Measurement of cardiac output in man using the technique of catheterization of the right auricle or ventricle. J Clin Invest 1945;24:104–16.

25. Slawsky MT, Colucci WS, Gottlieb SS, et al. Acute hemodynamic and clinical effects of levosimendan in patients with severe heart failure. Study Investigators. Circulation 2000;102(18):2222–7.

26. Abraham WT, Adams KF, Fonarow GC, et al. In-hospital mortality in patients with acute decompensated heart failure requiring intravenous vasoactive medications: an analysis from the Acute Decompensated Heart Failure National Registry (ADHERE). J Am Coll Cardiol 2005;46:57–64.

27. O'Connor CM, Gattis WA, Uretsky BF, et al. Continuous intravenous dobutamine is associated with an increased risk of death in patients with advanced heart failure: insights from the Flolan International Randomized Survival Trial (FIRST). Am Heart J 1999;138:78–86.

28. Cuffe MS, Califf RM, Adams KF Jr, et al. Short-term intravenous milrinone for acute exacerbation of chronic heart failure: a randomized controlled trial. JAMA 2002;287(12):1541–7.

29. William TA, Abraham K. Heart failure, CHAPTER 12 The Heart Failure Hospitalization. The McGraw-Hill companies; 2007. p. 147–69.

30. Russ MA, Prondzinsky R, Christoph A, et al. Hemodynamic improvement following levosimendan treatment in patients with acute myocardial infarction and cardiogenic shock. Crit Care Med 2007;35(12):2732–9.

31. Nanas JN, Papazoglou P, Tsagalou EP, et al. Efficacy and safety of intermittent, long-term, concomitant dobutamine and levosimendan infusions in severe heart failure refractory to dobutamine alone. Am J Cardiol 2005;95(6):768–71.

32. Scheidt S, Wilner G, Mueller H, et al. Intra-aortic balloon counterpulsation in cardiogenic shock. Report of a co-operative clinical trial. N Engl J Med 1973;288:979–84.

33. De Silva K, Lumley M, Kailey B, et al. Coronary and microvascular physiology during intra-aortic balloon counterpulsation. JACC Cardiovasc Interv 2014;7: 631–40.

34. Barron HV, Every NR, Parsons LS, et al. The use of intra-aortic balloon counterpulsation in patients with cardiogenic shock complicating acute myocardial infarction: data from the National Registry of Myocardial Infarction 2. Am Heart J 2001;141: 933–9.

35. Thiele H, Zeymer U, Neumann FJ, et al. Intraaortic balloon support for myocardial infarction with cardiogenic shock. N Engl J Med 2012;367: 1287–96.

36. Windecker S, Kolh P, Alfonso F, et al. 2014 ESC/EACTS guidelines on myocardial revascularization: the task force on myocardial revascularization of the European Society of Cardiology (ESC) and the European Association for Cardio-Thoracic Surgery (EACTS)developed with the special contribution of the European Association of Percutaneous Cardiovascular Interventions (EAPCI). Eur Heart J 2014; 35:2541–619.

37. van Nunen LX, van 't Veer M, Schampaert S, et al. Intra-aortic balloon counterpulsation reduces mortality in large anterior myocardial infarction complicated by persistent ischaemia: a CRISP-AMI substudy. EuroIntervention 2015;11:286–92.

38. Shah M, Patnaik S, Patel B, et al. Trends in mechanical circulatory support use and hospital mortality among patients with acute myocardial infarction and non-infarction related cardiogenic shock in the United States. Clin Res Cardiol 2018;107: 287–303.

39. Rathod KS, Koganti S, Iqbal MB, et al. Contemporary trends in cardiogenic shock: Incidence, intra-aortic balloon pump utilisation and outcomes from the London Heart Attack Group. Eur Heart J Acute Cardiovasc Care 2018;7:16–27.

40. Kolobow T, Spragg RG, Pierce JE, et al. Extended term (to 16 days) partial extracorporeal blood gas exchange with the spiral membrane lung in unanesthetized lambs. Trans Am Soc Artif Intern Organs 1971;17:350–4.

41. UK Collaborative ECMO Trial Group UK collaborative randomised trial of neonatal extracorporeal membrane oxygenation. UK Collaborative ECMO Trail Group. Lancet 1996;348:75–82.

42. Zapol WM, Snider MT, Hill JD, et al. Extracorporeal membrane oxygenation in severe acute respiratory failure. A randomized prospective study. JAMA 1979;242:2193–6.

43. Ahn C, Kim W, Cho Y, et al. Efficacy of extracorporeal cardiopulmonary resuscitation compared to conventional cardiopulmonary resuscitation for adult cardiac arrest patients: a systematic review and meta-analysis. Sci Rep 2016;6:34208.

44. Mitsui N, Koyama T, Marui A, et al. Experience with emergency cardiac surgery following institution of percutaneous cardiopulmonary support. Artif Organs 1999;23:496–9.

45. Rubino A, Costanzo D, Stanszus D, et al. Central veno-arterial extracorporeal membrane oxygenation (C-VA-ECMO) after cardiothoracic surgery: a single-center experience. J Cardiothorac Vasc Anesth 2018;32:1169–74.

46. Sakamoto T, Morimura N, Nagao K, et al. Extracorporeal cardiopulmonary resuscitation versus conventional cardiopulmonary resuscitation in adults with out-of-hospital cardiac arrest: a prospective observational study. Resuscitation 2014;85:762–8.

47. Aiba T, Nonogi H, Itoh T, et al. Appropriate indications for the use of a percutaneous cardiopulmonary support system in cases with cardiogenic shock complicating acute myocardial infarction. Jpn Circ J 2001;65:145–9.

48. Yonezu K, Sakakura K, Watanabe Y, et al. Determinants of survival and favorable neurologic outcomes in ischemic heart disease treated by veno-arterial extracorporeal membrane oxygenation. Heart Vessels 2018;33:25–32.

49. Repessé X, Au SM, Bréchot N, et al. Recombinant factor VIIa for uncontrollable bleeding in patients with extracorporeal membrane oxygenation: report on 15 cases and literature review. Crit Care 2013; 17:R55.

50. Muehrcke DD, McCarthy PM, Stewart RW, et al. Complications of extracorporeal life support systems using heparin-bound surfaces. The risk of intracardiac clot formation. J Thorac Cardiovasc Surg 1995;110:843–51.

51. Kern MJ. The changing paradigm of hemodynamic support device selection for high-risk percutaneous coronary interventions. J Invasive Cardiol 2011;23: 439–46.

52. Watanabe S, Fish K, Kovacic JC, et al. Left ventricular unloading using an impella CP improves coronary flow and infarct zone perfusion in ischemic heart failure. J Am Heart Assoc 2018;7:e006462.

53. O'Neill WW. A prospective, randomized clinical trial of hemodynamic support with Impella 2.5 versus intra-aortic balloon pump in patients undergoing high-risk percutaneous coronary intervention: the PROTECT II study. Circulation 2012;126:1717–22.

54. O'Neill WW, Schreiber T, Wohns DH, et al. The current use of Impella 2.5 in acute myocardial infarction complicated by cardiogenic shock: results from the USpella Registry. J Interv Cardiol 2014;27:1–11.

55. Engström AE, Sjauw KD, Baan J, et al. Long-term safety and sustained left ventricular recovery: long-term results of percutaneous left ventricular support with Impella LP2.5 in ST-elevation myocardial infarction. EuroIntervention 2011;6:860–5.

56. Griffith BP, Anderson MB, Samuels LE, et al. The RECOVER I: a multicenter prospective study of Impella 5.0/LD for postcardiotomy circulatory support. J Thorac Cardiovasc Surg 2013;145:548–54.

57. Seyfarth M, Sibbing D, Bauer I, et al. A randomized clinical trial to evaluate the safety and efficacy of a percutaneous left ventricular assist device versus intra-aortic balloon pumping for treatment of cardiogenic shock caused by myocardial infarction. J Am Coll Cardiol 2008;52:1584–8.

58. Ouweneel DM, Eriksen E, Sjauw KD, et al. Percutaneous mechanical circulatory support versus intra-aortic balloon pump in cardiogenic shock after acute myocardial infarction. J Am Coll Cardiol 2017;69:278–87.

59. Flaherty MP, Khan AR, O'Neill WW. Early initiation of impella in acute myocardial infarction complicated by cardiogenic shock improves survival: a meta-analysis. JACC Cardiovasc Interv 2017;10: 1805–6.

60. Pappalardo F, Schulte C, Pieri M, et al. Concomitant implantation of Impella® on top of veno-arterial extracorporeal membrane oxygenation may improve survival of patients with cardiogenic shock. Eur J Heart Fail 2017;19:404–12.

61. Patel SM, Lipinski J, Al-Kindi SG, et al. Simultaneous venoarterial extracorporeal membrane oxygenation and percutaneous left ventricular decompression therapy with Impella is associated with improved outcomes in refractory cardiogenic shock. ASAIO J 2019;65:21–8.

62. Thiele H, Sick P, Boudriot E, et al. Randomized comparison of intra-aortic balloon support with a percutaneous left ventricular assist device in patients with revascularized acute myocardial infarction complicated by cardiogenic shock. Eur Heart J 2005;26: 1276–83.

Acute Decompensated Heart Failure in Patients with Heart Failure with Reduced Ejection Fraction

Mitsuhiro Fukata, MD, PhD

KEYWORDS

- Acute decompensated heart failure • Heart failure with reduced ejection fraction (HFrEF)
- Decompensation • Heart failure treatment • Mechanical circulatory support

KEY POINTS

- Almost half of all hospitalized patients with heart failure are diagnosed with heart failure with reduced ejection fraction.
- Treatment strategy for acute decompensated heart failure depends on the fluid volume and perfusion status of end-organ systems.
- Drug titration and mechanical circulatory support devices should be considered for patients with acute decompensated heart failure with reduced ejection fraction.
- Sacubitril-valsartan therapy and/or dapagliflozin are new promising treatments for acute decompensated heart failure with reduced ejection fraction.

INTRODUCTION

Acute decompensated heart failure (ADHF) is a condition with new or worsening heart failure symptoms. The symptoms of heart failure often worsen rapidly and patients have frequent emergency visits hospitalizations. This unstable condition requires immediate treatments because it impairs perfusion to systemic organs and their function. Underlying disorder varies widely. Half of all patients with ADHF are diagnosed heart failure with reduced left ventricular ejection fraction (HFrEF). A few patients with ADHF with HFrEF present with cardiogenic shock. Many patients with HFrEF have a favorable response to treatments, but some patients continue to remain at risk for recurrence. Because the progression of heart failure disease, including episodes during hospitalization, can further worsen prognosis, appropriate drug titration and careful follow-ups are necessary to improve survival outcomes.

MECHANISM OF COMPENSATION IN HEART FAILURE WITH REDUCED LEFT VENTRICULAR EJECTION FRACTION AND ITS DETERIORATION

Almost half of all patients with decompensated heart failure were reported as HFrEF.[1,2] The changes in hemodynamics after a sudden-onset left ventricle (LV) dysfunction include (1) the temporary effect of deteriorated LV systolic function, (2) subsequent compensation by the sympathetic nervous system and renin-angiotensin-aldosterone system (RAAS; **Fig. 1**), and (3) chronic compensations resulting from partial LV functional recovery and renal retention of fluid.[3] In HFrEF (left ventricle ejection fraction [LVEF] <40%),[4] the volume retention is one of the

Department of Hematology, Oncology and Cardiovascular Medicine, Heart Center, Kyushu University Hospital, 3-1-1 Maidashi, Higashi-ku, Fukuoka 812-8582, Japan
E-mail address: mfukata-circ@umin.net

Heart Failure Clin 16 (2020) 187–200
https://doi.org/10.1016/j.hfc.2019.12.007
1551-7136/20/© 2019 Elsevier Inc. All rights reserved.

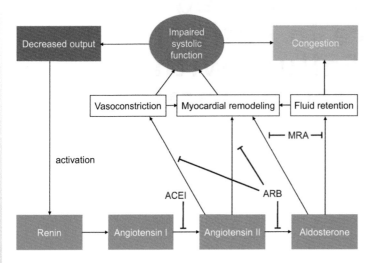

Fig. 1. Pathophysiologic role of the RAAS and its inhibitors in patients with HFrEF. Released renin cleaves angiotensin I from angiotensinogen. Angiotensin I is converted to angiotensin II by angiotensin-converting enzyme. Angiotensin II induces vasoconstriction, myocardial remodeling, and aldosterone secretion. Aldosterone also provokes myocardial remodeling and promotes volume retention via reabsorption of sodium in kidney. Angiotensin-converting enzyme inhibitor (ACEI) blocks conversion of angiotensin I to II. Angiotensin receptor blocker (ARB) blocks vasoconstriction and myocardial remodeling by angiotensin II. Mineralocorticoid receptor antagonist (MRA) blocks myocardial remodeling and fluid retention by aldosterone.

compensated mechanisms that maintain a certain amount of cardiac output. The recovery phase, in which volume retention augments cardiac output, is called compensated heart failure. However, the heart may not be able to increase cardiac output to meet the oxygenation demands from end organs and peripheral circulation, especially if LV systolic dysfunction is present.[5]

If the heart becomes severely damaged, compensation by the sympathetic nervous reflexes and activated RAAS, as well as fluid retention in the heart, is not able to produce a normal cardiac output.[6] Decreased cardiac output continues to increase the sympathetic nerve activities and activate the RAAS, subsequently regulating the heart rate, blood pressure, and blood volume fluid balance (see **Fig. 1**). A continued activation of these neurohumoral systems eventually results in an exacerbation of heart failure.[7,8] The poor cardiac output leads to progressive retention of blood volume fluid, causing progressive increase of the systemic filling pressure and the right atrial pressure. The excessive volume retention provides an increase in LV end-diastolic pressure (LVEDP), resulting in pulmonary congestion, which can cause further impairment of cardiac function. This condition is called decompensated heart failure. Clinically, the condition of decompensation is detected by the manifestation of progressive systemic and pulmonary edema, and/or end-organ dysfunction from systemic hypoperfusion. Inappropriate therapy at this stage may lead to life-threatening events.

HEMODYNAMICS AND SYMPTOMATIC PRESENTATION IN ACUTE DECOMPENSATED HEART FAILURE

The events of acute decompensation in patients with chronic heart failure can be triggered by 1 or more factors, such as infection, uncontrolled hypertension, dysrhythmia, or noncompliance with medications and diet. The risk factors for ADHF are shown in **Box 1**. There are 3 common modes of onset: (1) acute cardiogenic pulmonary edema, (2) systemic fluid retention, and (3) hypoperfusion caused by low cardiac output, which is under clinical scenario (CS) 1 to 3 (**Table 1**).[9] CS 1 signifies a condition that presents with acute pulmonary edema by central volume shift with systemic blood pressure more than 140 mm Hg. CS 1 accounts for approximately 10% of ADHF.[10] CS 2 represents a condition that presents with systemic edema and mild pulmonary edema with chronic increase of LVEDP. Systemic blood pressure in CS 2 patients is in the range of 100 to 140 mm Hg. CS 3 is a condition that presents with systemic hypoperfusion with mild volume retention and mild pulmonary edema. Systemic blood pressure in the CS 3 is less than 100 mm Hg. Hypotension as a consequence of hypoperfusion is likely secondary to LV systolic dysfunction because it cannot adequately respond to the preload.

The symptoms of congestion present with a rapid increase in LVEDP.[11] As the left atrial pressure increases, patients experience fatigue and exercise intolerance.[5] Bendopnea is a recently reported novel symptom in patients with heart failure, defined as a shortness of breath when bending forward, such as when tying shoelaces or putting on socks.[12] Trepopnea is a shortness of breath that is experienced in the lateral decubitus position on 1 side but not on the other, recognized in patients with heart failure.[13,14] When it is further decompensated, symptoms can be observed even at rest, such as paroxysmal nocturnal dyspnea. Acute pulmonary edema is associated with venous reservoirs. Recurrent episodes of hypoxemia and sudden increase in

---

Box 1
Exacerbation factors for heart failure

Ischemic heart disease (acute coronary syndrome, chronic myocardial ischemia)

Tachyarrhythmia (atrial fibrillation, atrial flutter, ventricular tachycardia, frequent premature ventricular contraction)

Bradyarrhythmia (atrioventricular block, sick sinus syndrome)

Valvular heart disease (exacerbation of mitral regurgitation or aortic stenosis)

Pericardial disease (constrictive pericarditis with or without pericardial effusion, cardiac tamponade)

Atriovenous fistula

Infection (pneumonia, infective endocardium, sepsis)

Hypertension

Anemia

Renal dysfunction

Adherence failure (saline restriction, water restriction, compliance with medication)

Acute pulmonary thromboembolism

Acute exacerbation of chronic obstructive pulmonary disease

Drugs (NSAIDs, drugs with negative inotropic effects, cancer chemotherapy)

Excessive physical or mental stress

Overwork

Hormonal and metabolic abnormalities (hyperthyroidism, adrenal dysfunction, peripartum cardiomyopathy)

Mechanical complications (cardiac rupture, acute mitral regurgitation, chest trauma, acute aortic dissection)

Abbreviation: NSAIDs, nonsteroidal antiinflammatory drugs.

---

afterload continue to activate the sympathetic nervous system and the other neurohumoral factors; this results in a sudden fluid redistribution. Pulmonary edema is further exacerbated by vasoconstriction in the highly compliant systemic venous reservoir through increase in LV preload. The pathophysiology of fluid retention is the vasoconstriction of renal arteries causing reduction in glomerular filtration rate by the activated sympathetic nervous system.[15] In addition, an activation of neurohumoral factors leads to reabsorption of water and sodium reuptake,[16] resulting in an increase in extracellular fluid volume and edema. This excessive fluid volume leads to end-organ dysfunction, so careful follow-ups are mandatory even if precise evaluations for edematous changes have not been established in the clinical setting.

In hospitalized patients with HFrEF, systolic blood pressure less than 130 mm Hg is associated with poor outcomes.[17] ADHF with low blood pressure includes cardiogenic shock or advanced phase of heart failure. In cardiogenic shock, circulatory failure also diminishes coronary blood supply and further decreases systolic function during the course of shock. This process may turn into a vicious cycle of cardiac deterioration if the coronary arteries continue to have poor perfusion. In cardiogenic shock caused by myocardial infarction, the coronary vessel flow is further reduced by preexisting coronary vessel blockages; even a small decrease in arterial pressure can set off a vicious cycle of cardiac deterioration. Thus, treating myocardial infarction is extremely important to prevent detrimental outcomes in the state of shock.

INITIAL ASSESSMENT FOR ACUTE DECOMPENSATED HEART FAILURE

ADHF can rapidly shift to cardiogenic shock or cardiopulmonary arrest. If the patient is in cardiopulmonary arrest at the time of arrival to the hospital, advanced cardiac life support is mandatory. The first step is to identify the cause of cardiogenic shock and respiratory failure. It is preferable to transport those patients to the nearest hospital equipped with a coronary care unit or intensive care unit where advanced cardiovascular care is available in cases that involve severe pulmonary

Table 1
Clinical scenarios in acute heart failure syndrome

Clinical Scenario	Characteristics
CS 1	SBP >140 mm Hg Symptoms develop abruptly Predominantly diffuse pulmonary edema Minimal systemic edema (patient may be euvolemic or hypovolemic) Acute elevation of filling pressure often with preserved LVEF Vascular pathophysiology
CS 2	SBP 100~140 mm Hg Symptoms develop gradually, together with a gradual increase in body weight Predominantly systemic edema Minimal pulmonary edema Chronic elevation of filling pressure, including increased venous pressure and elevated pulmonary arterial pressure Manifestations of organ dysfunction (renal impairment, liver dysfunction, anemia, hypoalbuminemia)
CS 3	SBP <100 mm Hg Rapid or gradual onset of symptoms Predominantly signs of hypoperfusion Minimal systemic and pulmonary edema Elevation of filling pressure Two subsets: Clear hypoperfusion or cardiogenic shock No hypoperfusion/cardiogenic shock
CS 4	Symptoms and signs of acute heart failure Evidence of ACS Isolated elevation of cardiac troponin is inadequate for CS4 classification
CS 5	Rapid or gradual onset No pulmonary edema Right ventricular dysfunction Signs of systemic venous congestion

Abbreviations: ACS, acute coronary syndrome; LVEF, left ventricular ejection fraction; SBP, systolic blood pressure.
Reprinted from Mebazaa A, et al.[9]

edema or cardiogenic shock.[18,19] The accurate diagnosis of acute heart failure and its cause should be attained by obtaining the history, such as prior hospitalizations related to heart failure, medications, past medical history, and appropriate physical examinations including vital signs and heart sounds.[20] It is important to exclude acute coronary syndrome and acute pulmonary thromboembolism because these diseases can be lethal but are reversible with early intervention. Echocardiography can be helpful to support the diagnosis of HFrEF and understand underlying structural abnormalities. In addition, high sensitivity and specificity of detecting pulmonary edema by lung echocardiography, even compared with B lines in chest radiographs, were reported.[21,22] Specific findings in physical examinations or B-type natriuretic peptide level are useful for differentiating noncardiogenic pulmonary edema.[23,24]

Therapeutic intervention should be performed at an early stage to stabilize patients' hemodynamics and respiratory status. Along with the diagnosis of

ADHF, the treatment strategy is determined according to the CS classification (see **Box 1**),[9] Nohria and colleagues'[25] classification, and pathologic classification.[20] For cardiogenic shock, change in lactic acid level is important to assess current perfusion status. Urine output should be also monitored as a marker of renal circulation.

TREATMENT STRATEGY FOR ACUTE DECOMPENSATED HEART FAILURE

Treatment guidelines from the American College of Cardiology (ACC)/American Heart Association (AHA) and European Society of Cardiology (ESC) differentiate ADHF management from chronic heart failure management.[4,26] The immediate goal of treatment of patients with ADHF is to improve symptoms and hemodynamics. Patients with acute heart failure who have percutaneous arterial oxygen saturation (SpO$_2$) less than 90% or arterial oxygen partial pressure (Pao$_2$) less than 60 mm Hg should be treated with supplemental oxygen. If respiratory rate is greater than

25 breaths/min or SpO$_2$ less than 90% under oxygen therapy, patients should be started on noninvasive positive airway pressure devices or considered to undergo endotracheal intubation.[4,27] The initial phase of treatment depends largely on patients' volume and perfusion status. Hence, it is recommended to classify patients who are hospitalized for symptoms of heart failure into 4 basic hemodynamic subtypes.[25,28] A patient with adequate perfusion and with congestion (warm and wet) should receive vasodilator and/or diuretics. A patient with adequate perfusion but without congestion (warm and dry) should be titrated with oral heart failure drugs. For instance, if blood pressure is not too low in "warm" patients, an angiotensin-converting enzyme inhibitor should be given or its dose should be increased. Patients with hypoperfusion and without congestion (cold and dry) should receive intravenous fluid at first to resuscitate the hypovolemic state; if the patient continues to remain decompensated, the use of ionotropic agents is recommended. Patients with hypoperfusion and congestion (cold and wet) should be treated with inotropic agent and mechanical circulatory support, especially if refractory to medications.

Once the patient's hemodynamic stability has been achieved in the initial phase of ADHF treatment, it is important to titrate drugs for heart failure and consider device therapy that is appropriate for relevant pathophysiology. It is also essential to continuously evaluate the patient's symptoms, vital signs, jugular venous distention, heart and respiratory sounds, leg edema, changes in body weight, fluid balance, and renal and liver function daily to make adequate corrections to ongoing treatments. If refractory to the initial treatments, other possible disorders should be considered, such as arrhythmia; valvular dysfunction, including valve destruction, caused by infective endocarditis should be appropriately diagnosed by close patient monitoring. Arterial pressure monitoring should be considered, especially when hemodynamics are unstable. Accurate hemodynamic measurements by Swan-Ganz catheter should be performed if the evaluation by the Nohria-Stevenson classification is considered to be insufficient; however, the routine use of Swan-Ganz catheters is not recommended.[29,30]

In patients with HFrEF, renin-angiotensin inhibitors and β-blockers should be started and increased to the target dose (**Fig. 2**, **Table 2**). β-Blocker therapy should be initiated once adequate perfusion, such as sufficient urine output and stable blood pressure, is achieved. Ivabradine should be considered in patients with symptomatic HFrEF in sinus rhythm with a resting heart rate more than 70 beats per minute (bpm) despite treatment with a sufficient dose of β-blockers because it reduces the combined end point of mortality or heart failure hospitalization in patients with symptomatic HFrEF in sinus rhythm and with a heart rate more than 70 bpm who had been hospitalized for heart failure (**Fig. 3**).[31] There are 2 randomized controlled trials that tested for new oral drug treatments for HFrEF. First, the administration of sacubitril-valsartan to patients with HFrEF was shown to reduce cardiovascular death and heart failure hospitalization compared with enalapril (see **Fig. 3**).[32] Even in ADHF, N-terminal pro–B-type natriuretic peptide (NT-proBNP) concentrations in patients with sacubitril-valsartan were significantly reduced compared with enalapril.[33] Second, dapagliflozin significantly reduced the risk of death or aggravation of heart failure compared with placebo in patients with HFrEF, regardless of the presence or absence of diabetes, even in older patients (see **Fig. 3**).[34,35] For patients at high risk for sudden

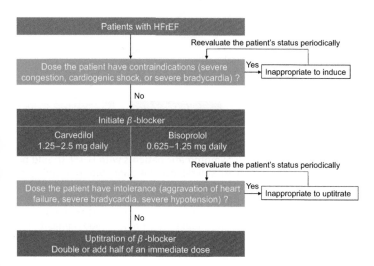

Fig. 2. Algorithm for induction and uptitration of β-blocker in patients with HFrEF. In symptomatic patients with HFrEF, induction of β-blocker is strongly recommended. To induce β-blocker, physicians have to evaluate contraindications and intolerability for the drug in each patient.

Table 2
Target dose of drugs for heart failure with reduced left ventricular ejection fraction

	Target Dose (mg/d)
Angiotensin-converting Enzyme Inhibitor	
Ramipril	5
Enalapril	10
Angiotensin Receptor Blocker	
Candesartan	16
Losartan	50
Valsartan	160
β-Blocker	
Carvedilol	25
Bisoprolol	5
Mineralocorticoid Receptor Antagonist	
Spironolactone	25
Eplerenone	25
Canrenone	50

cardiac events related to ventricular arrhythmia (ie, LVEF<35%, prominent heart failure symptoms, frequent nonsustained ventricular tachycardia), implantation of an implantable cardioverter-defibrillator should be considered. Patients with wide QRS duration and low LVEF should also be considered for cardiac resynchronization therapy. Other comorbidities that can affect heart failure should also be diagnosed and the patients started on treatments if necessary. The comorbidities to be treated include cardiac disorders (ie, atrial fibrillation,[36,37] ventricular arrhythmia,[38] ischemic heart disease,[39] valvular heart disease,[40] cardiac amyloidosis[41]) or noncardiac conditions (ie, hypertension,[42] iron deficiency,[43] depressive state[44]). In addition, physical rehabilitation in older patients who were hospitalized for ADHF showed improvements in physical function and reduction in rehospitalizations.[45]

INTRAVENOUS DRUGS
Inotropic Agents

Inotropic drugs, such as dobutamine and milrinone, may initially help to stabilize hemodynamic

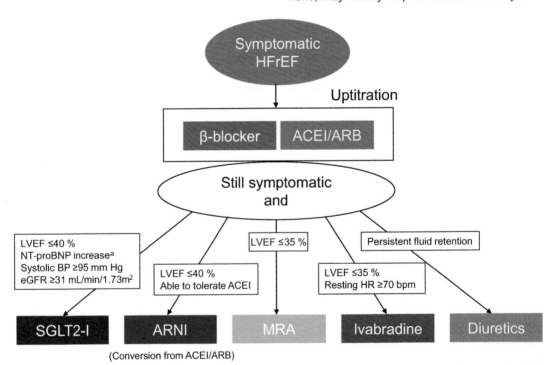

Fig. 3. Treatment algorithm for symptomatic patients with HFrEF. Symptomatic patients with HFrEF should be generally have β-blocker and ACEI or ARB induced. Patients who are still symptomatic and with reduced ejection fraction despite the uptitrated dose are candidates for sodium glucose cotransporter 2 inhibitor (SGLT2-I), angiotensin receptor-neprilysin inhibitor (ARNI), MRA, ivabradine, and diuretics. Compatibility for these drugs is evaluated according to the specific condition in clinical trials, as described here. [a] N-terminal pro–B-type natriuretic peptide (NT-proBNP) concentration greater than or equal to 600 pg/mL (≥400 pg/mL if hospitalized for HF within the previous 12 months, ≥900 pg/mL in patients with atrial fibrillation or atrial flutter). HR, heart rate.

derangements. Patients who need these drugs may not tolerate β-blocker therapy initially. Drugs with cardiotonic effects are also indicated for patients with hypotension or peripheral circulatory failure, as well as patients who are resistant to fluid resuscitation. Cardiotonic medications are often used for patients with LV enlargement and reduced LVEF; however, they increase myocardial oxygen demand and induce myocardial calcium load, resulting in arrhythmia, myocardial ischemia, and/or myocardial injury. Thus, a prolonged use of these drugs is not recommended because they may increase mortality. The Acutely Decompensated Heart Failure National Registry (ADHERE) study showed a higher in-hospital mortality in patients who received cardiotonic drugs than in those who received vasodilators, even after correcting for blood pressure.[2] Thus, the indication of inotropic drugs and administration period should be determined carefully.

Dobutamine is a recombinant catecholamine. In addition to positive inotropic effects, it has mild vasodilatory effects that cause a decrease in systemic peripheral vascular resistance and pulmonary capillary pressure at a dosage of 5 μg/kg/min or less. Compared with other catecholamines, dobutamine causes less myocardial oxygen consumption, consequently it is used as a preferred drug in the setting of ischemic heart disease. Dobutamine reduces pulmonary diastolic pressure and is effective in reducing pulmonary congestion. In patients on carvedilol for the treatment of chronic heart failure, the effect of increasing cardiac output is reported to be diminished.[46] An analysis of the FIRST (Flolan International Randomized Survival Trial) study has shown the possibility of increasing the incidence of cardiac events by dobutamine,[47] thus, it is desirable to limit its use to the minimum dose and the shortest administration period.

Milrinone is a phosphodiesterase (PDE) inhibitor that strengthens myocardial contractility by increasing cyclic adenosine monophosphate levels and protein kinase A activity, and promoting intracellular calcium entry. In patients with heart failure who receive a β-blocker, the inotropic effect by dobutamine or dopamine is limited because the sympathetic receptor is blocked, whereas PDE inhibitors that can act besides the sympathetic signaling pathway are potentially more effective than catecholamine. Milrinone increased cardiac output and reduced pulmonary capillary pressure without significant heart rate change.[48] According to the analysis of the ADHERE study, the in-hospital prognosis of patients with heart failure receiving milrinone was better than that of patients with heart failure receiving dobutamine by pairwise comparison.[2] However, milrinone-treated patients had more sustained hypotension requiring intervention and new atrial arrhythmias compared with placebo-treated patients in the Outcomes of a Prospective Trial of Intravenous Milrinone for Exacerbations of Chronic Heart Failure (OPTIME-CHF) study.[49] Therefore, routine use of intravenous milrinone is not recommended.

Dopamine is an endogenous catecholamine and is a precursor of noradrenaline. At low dosages (<2 μg/kg/min), it has a diuretic effect via renal artery dilation and direct action on renal tubules.[50] At moderate dosages (2–10 μg/kg/min), β1 receptor stimulation, increased noradrenalin release from the heart and peripheral blood vessels, and α1 receptor stimulation cause positive inotropic effects, resulting in increased heart rates and systemic vascular resistance. At high dosages (10–20 μg/kg/min), the effect on the α1 receptor becomes predominant and vascular resistance further increases. Physiologically, dopamine could be suitable for acute heart failure with low blood pressure in patients with HFrEF in the short term. In contrast, decrease in urine volume was observed in patients with ejection fraction greater than 50% in subgroup analysis of the Renal Optimization Strategies Evaluation (ROSE) study,[51] so the use of this drug depends on the condition of the patient.

Norepinephrine is an endogenous catecholamine that shows positive inotropic and chronotropic effects by stimulating β1 receptors. It can also act on α receptors to exert arterial vasoconstriction in the periphery. Patients with heart failure with sepsis are good candidates for this drug because infection-related release of vasodilatory mediators lead to reduce arterial resistance.[52,53] Although the mean arterial pressure increases from increased peripheral vascular resistance, norepinephrine increases afterload as well as myocardial oxygen consumption. It also decreases blood flow into the kidneys, brain, and intestines. Thus, it should only be used for a short period. For patients who need to use high doses of norepinephrine to maintain blood pressure and organ perfusion, a mechanical device for circulation support, such as intra-aortic balloon pump (IABP) or venoarterial extracorporeal membrane oxygenation (VA-ECMO), should be considered in order to reduce noradrenaline dose.

Vasodilators

Vasodilators (eg, nitrate, carperitide) are the first choice of medications in patients with acute heart failure with dyspnea caused by increased LVEDP and/or pulmonary edema with noncompromised peripheral circulation. Vasodilators are especially desirable for patients with high blood pressure (representatively >140 mm Hg), myocardial ischemia, and mitral regurgitation. The use of calcium antagonists is not recommended in the treatment of ADHF with recued LVEF because it could aggravate heart failure.[54] Because excessive blood pressure reduction may decrease renal function, it is important to periodically measure serum creatinine level during the administration of vasodilators. In particular, patients with preexisting renal dysfunction, older age, or aortic valve stenosis have a higher risk for acute renal failure.

Nitrate stimulates guanylate cyclase in vascular smooth muscle cells via nitrogen monoxide, dilating venous capacity vessels at low doses and arterial resistance vessels at high doses. Nitrate decreases pulmonary capillary pressure but increases cardiac output by increasing preload and decreasing afterload. Patients with heart failure with ischemic heart disease receive benefit from nitrate by the effect of coronary artery dilation.

Diuretics

Loop diuretics alleviate the symptoms of heart failure by improving pulmonary congestion, pleural effusion, and edema in extremities. This process occurs by reducing preload and decreasing left ventricular end-diastolic pressure. In patients with ADHF, the effect is generally immediate.[55] In an observational study, the early treatment cases in which furosemide was administered less than 60 minutes after arrival had a low in-hospital mortality independent of other confounding factors.[56] Thus, early administration of furosemide should be considered for ADHF with preserved circulatory state. Patients with severe heart failure often have associated acute or acute-on-chronic renal dysfunction. In these patients, tubular secretion of furosemide is decreased, so they require a higher dose than usual.[57] Continuous intravenous administration is sometimes superior in diuretic effect to bolus intravenous administration.[58] In the Diuretic Optimization Strategies Evaluation (DOSE) study,[59] although the proportion of patients with exacerbation of renal function was greater in patients with high-dose intravenous administration of loop diuretics than in patients with low-dose loop diuretics, no significant differences were detected in heart failure symptom improvement and survival time between the 2 groups. Therefore, generally, the dose of loop diuretics should be minimized. It has been reported that the effects of this drug may be different in LVEF,[60] and it is necessary to examine

the dosage according to the pathologic condition. In patients with acidosis, hypotension, hyponatremia, and hypoalbuminemia, the response from diuretic drugs was poor. In order to improve the effect of diuresis, adding another agent with different sites of action, such as thiazide or mineralocorticoid receptor antagonists, can be effective.[61,62]

Tolvaptan is an oral drug that inhibits the arginine vasopressin type 2 receptor. In a randomized controlled trial with placebo (Efficacy of Vasopressin Antagonism in Heart Failure Outcome Study With Tolvaptan (EVEREST) study), tolvaptan improved congestive symptoms; however, long-term prognosis was not changed.[63,64] In Japan, it has been used in patients with heart failure who are resistant to other diuretics. Although the improvement of fluid retention was shown in Targeting Acute Congestion With Tolvaptan in Congestive Heart Failure (TACTICS-HF) and Study to Evaluate Challenging Responders to Therapy in Congestive Heart Failure (SECRET-CHF) studies, symptom-reducing effects of tolvaptan were limited.[65,66] Therefore, it is considered effective for patients with severe congestive symptoms who are refractory to conventional diuretic use. Its side effects include hypernatremia, especially in older patients, subsequently requiring close monitoring. Rapid increase in serum sodium level in patients with chronic hyponatremia may lead to central pontine myelinolysis, a potentially fatal and debilitating neurologic condition. Thus, after the induction of tolvaptan, serum sodium level is recommended to be measured at 4 to 6 hours and 8 to 12 hours after administration, followed by daily measurement for several days after administration. If serum sodium levels increase above the normal range, immediate discontinuation of tolvaptan and hydration, including infusion of 5% sugar solution, should be considered.

MECHANICAL CIRCULATORY SUPPORT FOR ACUTE DECOMPENSATED HEART FAILURE IN PATIENTS WITH HEART FAILURE WITH REDUCED EJECTION FRACTION
Intra-aortic Balloon Pump

The mechanism of IABP circulatory support is to reduce cardiac workload by reducing afterload and to improve myocardial oxygenation by enhancing coronary blood flow by means of counterpulsation of a balloon placed in the descending aorta. It is recommended to start mechanical circulatory support in patients with ADHF and patients with HFrEF with end-organ malperfusion despite volume optimization and

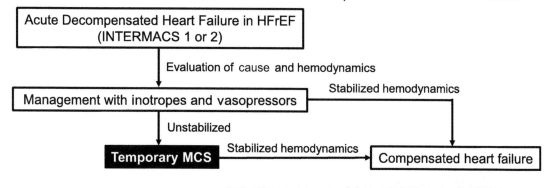

	IABP	VA-ECMO	Impella 5.0	TandemHeart
Support flow (L/min)	0.2–1.0	2.5–7.0	1.0–5.0	2.5–5.0
Working chamber	Ao	RA → Ao	LV → Ao	LA → Ao
Maximum implant duration	5–7 d	3–4 wk	2 wk	2 wk
LV filling pressure (LVEDP)	↓	↑ or ↑↑	↓↓	↓↓
LV afterload	↓	↑↑↑	↓↓	↓↓
Coronary perfusion	↑↑	→ or ↑	↑	↑
Peripheral perfusion	↑	↑↑	↑↑	↑↑
Oxygenation	—	Possible	—	Possible

Fig. 4. Mechanical circulatory support in acute decompensation in HFrEF. The treatment strategy for severe cardiogenic shock or progressive decline (INTERMACS profile 1 or 2) is shown in the upper flowchart. Properties of each device are listed below. Ao; aorta; HFrEF, heart failure with reduced ejection fraction; IABP, intra-aortic balloon pumping; INTERMACS, interagency registry for mechanically assisted circulatory support; LV, left ventricle; LVEDP, left ventricular end-diastolic pressure; MCS, mechanical circulatory support; RA, right atrium; VA-ECMO, veno-arterial extra-corporeal membranous oxygenation.

requiring more than 1 catecholamine support (Interagency Registry for Mechanically Assisted Circulatory Support [INTERMACS] profile 1 or 2; **Fig. 4, Table 3**). Patients with heart failure with ischemic heart disease or mitral regurgitation are more likely to benefit from the use of these devices as well. However, the use of IABP has not improved the prognosis of cardiogenic shock secondary to acute myocardial infarction (IABP-SHOCK II trial).[67,68] Therefore, the routine use of these devices is not recommended. The assist effect is attenuated when the patient also has arrhythmia or severe and persistent tachycardia. Contraindications to the use of IABP include moderate or higher aortic regurgitation and aortic dissection. Lower limb ischemia on the side of balloon insertion, hemorrhages, aortic dissection, infection, and thrombosis are commonly reported complications.

Venoarterial Extracorporeal Membrane Oxygenation

VA-ECMO is a cardiopulmonary assist device consisting of centrifugal pump and extracorporeal oxygenator that can be percutaneously inserted.

It is also used for patients in ADHF with reduced ejection fraction and poor circulation despite volume optimization and catecholamine/vasopressor use (INTERMACS profile 1 or 2; see **Fig. 4, Table 3**). Peripheral VA-ECMO is classically accomplished through the femoral artery and vein. The assisting flow is affected by the size and position of the cannulation. If cardiac function is not sufficiently recovered after the use of peripheral VA-ECMO, or if it is considered difficult to continue because of complications such as bleeding, central approach for ECMO (suction at right atrium, discharge ascending aorta) is an option to maintain stable circulatory assistance. The survival rate after VA-ECMO is 25% to 60% for cardiogenic shock.[69,70] Simultaneous use of IABP with VA-ECMO is reasonable because IABP can partially offset afterload increased by VA-ECMO and can provide coronary flow augmentation (see **Fig. 4**). In a meta-analysis, the use of concomitant IABP in patients with VA-ECMO did not change mortality in the total population but was associated with lower mortality in patients with acute myocardial infarction compared with patients with VA-ECMO alone.[71]

Table 3
Interagency Registry for Mechanically Assisted Circulatory Support profiles

Level	Condition	Suggested MCS	Time to MCS
1	Critical cardiogenic shock. "Crash and burn" Hemodynamic instability in spite of increasing doses of catecholamines and/or mechanical circulatory support with critical hypoperfusion of target organs. NYHA IV	Percutaneous support device including IABP and VA-ECMO, Extracorporeal LVAD	Within hours
2	Progressive decline despite inotropic support "Sliding" on inotropes Intravenous inotropic support with acceptable blood pressure but rapid deterioration of renal function, nutritional state, or signs of congestion. NYHA IV	Percutaneous support device including IABP and VA-ECMO, extracorporeal LVAD, implantable LVAD	Within a few days
3	Stable but inotrope dependent. Dependent stability Hemodynamic stability with low or intermediate doses of inotropes, but necessary because of hypotension, worsening of symptoms, or progressive renal failure. NYHA IV	Implantable LVAD	Within a few weeks
4	Resting symptoms. "Frequent flyer" Temporary cessation of inotropic treatment, but patients present with frequent symptom recurrences and typically with fluid overload NYHA ambulatory IV	Implantable LVAD (especially in patients with frequent ICD therapy)	Within weeks to months
5	Exertion intolerant. Housebound Complete cessation of physical activity, stable at rest, but frequently with moderate fluid retention and some level of renal dysfunction. NYHA ambulatory IV	LVAD in patients with frequent ICD therapy	—
6	Exertion limited. "Walking wounded" Minor limitation on physical activity and absence of congestion while at rest. Easily fatigued by light activity. NYHA III	LVAD in patients with frequent ICD therapy	—
7	Advanced NYHA III. "Placeholder" NYHA class III with no current or recent unstable fluid balance	LVAD in patients with frequent ICD therapy	—

Abbreviations: IABP, intra-aortic balloon pump; ICD, implantable cardioverter-defibrillator; LVAD, left ventricular assist device; MCS, mechanical circulatory support; NYHA, New York Heart Association functional classification; VA-ECMO, venoarterial extracorporeal membrane oxygenation.
Adapted from Stevenson LW, et al.[76]

Impella

The Impella is a percutaneous left ventricular assist device with a pigtail-shaped tip, which is placed in the LV and delivers blood through the LV to ascending aorta anterogradely by an axial flow pump. The device can reduce the left ventricular pressure and volume, thus decreasing myocardial oxygen demand. From this mechanism of hemodynamic support, the device is considered to be particularly useful in acute myocardial infarction with shock and fulminant myocarditis. Cardiac power output (CPO) is an indicator of hemodynamics calculated as mean atrial pressure × cardiac output/451, and has a strong association with in-hospital mortality in patients with cardiogenic shock.[72] The CPO is an important parameter when using Impella in the management of severe heart failure.

TandemHeart

TandemHeart is also a percutaneous device that is placed in the left atrium bypassing the femoral artery, consisting of a transseptal cannula, arterial cannula, and a centrifugal blood pump. Clinical trials for this device have shown superior hemodynamic support compared with IABP in the setting of cardiogenic shock.[73,74] In the initiation process of this device, a venting cannula is placed in the left atrium through a transseptal puncture. Therefore, operators should have enough experience in this procedure.[75] After the removal of the device, an interatrial shunt resides until septal closure is performed.

SUMMARY

Because decompensated heart failure is a critical disease with a high mortality, therapy to improve patients' hemodynamics should be initiated immediately. Especially in HFrEF, extensive evidence and accumulated clinical experience support the management of the disease. Although the effectiveness of new drugs such as sodium glucose cotransporter 2 inhibitor or angiotensin receptor-neprilysin inhibitor has been shown, some patients with HFrEF are still at risk for recurrence of decompensated heart failure. Therefore, further development of treatment is still needed.

ACKNOWLEDGMENTS

The author would like to thank Rakushumimarika Harada for editing the article. This work was supported by JSPS KAKENHI grant number JP17K11577.

DISCLOSURE

The author has nothing to disclose.

REFERENCES

1. Hernandez AF, Hammill BG, O'Connor CM, et al. Clinical effectiveness of beta-blockers in heart failure: findings from the OPTIMIZE-HF (Organized Program to Initiate Lifesaving Treatment in Hospitalized Patients with Heart Failure) Registry. J Am Coll Cardiol 2009;5:184–92.
2. Abraham WT, Adams KF, Fonarow GC, et al. In-hospital mortality in patients with acute decompensated heart failure requiring intravenous vasoactive medications: an analysis from the Acute Decompensated Heart Failure National Registry (ADHERE). J Am Coll Cardiol 2005;46:57–64.
3. Hall JE. Guyton and hall textbook of medical physiology. 13th edition. :Amsterdam: Elsevier; 2015. p. 271–80.
4. Ponikowski P, Voors AA, Anker SD, et al. 2016 ESC guidelines for the diagnosis and treatment of acute and chronic heart failure: The Task Force for the diagnosis and treatment of acute and chronic heart failure of the European Society of Cardiology (ESC) Developed with the special contribution of the Heart Failure Association (HFA) of the ESC. Eur Heart J 2016;37:2129–200.
5. Del Buono MG, Arena R, Borlaug BA, et al. Exercise intolerance in patients with heart failure: JACC state-of-the-art review. J Am Coll Cardiol 2019;73: 2209–25.
6. Hartupee J, Mann DL. Neurohormonal activation in heart failure with reduced ejection fraction. Nat Rev Cardiol 2017;14:30–8.
7. Miller WL. Fluid volume overload and congestion in heart failure: time to reconsider pathophysiology and how volume is assessed. Circ Heart Fail 2016; 9:e002922.
8. Opie LH. Compensation and overcompensation in congestive heart failure. Am Heart J 1990;120(6 Pt 2):1552–7.
9. Mebazaa A, Gheorghiade M, Piña IL, et al. Practical recommendations for prehospital and early in-hospital management of patients presenting with acute heart failure syndromes. Crit Care Med 2008;36(1 Suppl):S129–39.
10. Nieminen MS, Brutsaert D, Dickstein K, et al. Euro-Heart Failure Survey II (EHFS II): a survey on hospitalized acute heart failure patients: description of population. Eur Heart J 2006;27:2725–36.
11. Ware LB, Matthay MA. Clinical practice. Acute pulmonary edema. N Engl J Med 2005;353:2788–96.
12. Thibodeau JT, Turer AT, Gualano SK, et al. Characterization of a novel symptom of advanced heart failure: bendopnea. JACC Heart Fail 2014;2:24–31.
13. Fujita M, Miyamoto S, Tambara K, et al. Trepopnea in patients with chronic heart failure. Int J Cardiol 2002; 84:115–8.
14. de Araujo BS, Reichert R, Eifer DA, et al. Trepopnea may explain right-sided pleural effusion in patients with decompensated heart failure. Am J Emerg Med 2012;30:925–31.e2.
15. Korner PI, Stokes GS, White SW, et al. Role of the autonomic nervous system in the renal vasoconstriction response to hemorrhage in the rabbit. Circ Res 1967;20:676–85.
16. DiBona GF, Zambraski EJ, Aguilera AJ, et al. Neurogenic control of renal tubular sodium reabsorption in the dog: a brief review and preliminary report concerning possible humoral mediation. Circ Res 1977;40(5 Suppl 1):I127–30.

17. Arundel C, Lam PH, Gill GS, et al. Systolic blood pressure and outcomes in patients with heart failure with reduced ejection fraction. J Am Coll Cardiol 2019;73:3054–63.

18. van Diepen S, Bakal JA, Lin M, et al. Variation in critical care unit admission rates and outcomes for patients with acute coronary syndromes or heart failure among high- and low-volume cardiac hospitals. J Am Heart Assoc 2015;4:e001708.

19. Shirakabe A, Kobayashi N, Okazaki H, et al. Trends in the management of acute heart failure requiring intensive care. Am J Cardiol 2019;124:1076–84.

20. Mebazaa A, Tolppanen H, Mueller C, et al. Acute heart failure and cardiogenic shock: a multidisciplinary practical guidance. Intensive Care Med 2016;42:147–63.

21. Picano E, Pellikka PA. Ultrasound of extravascular lung water: a new standard for pulmonary congestion. Eur Heart J 2016;37:2097–104.

22. Maw AM, Hassanin A, Ho PM, et al. Diagnostic accuracy of point-of-care lung ultrasonography and chest radiography in adults with symptoms suggestive of acute decompensated heart failure: a systematic review and meta-analysis. JAMA Netw Open 2019;2:e190703.

23. Renier W, Winckelmann KH, Verbakel JY, et al. Signs and symptoms in adult patients with acute dyspnea: a systematic review and meta-analysis. Eur J Emerg Med 2018;25:3–11.

24. Morrison LK, Harrison A, Krishnaswamy P, et al. Utility of a rapid B-natriuretic peptide assay in differentiating congestive heart failure from lung disease in patients presenting with dyspnea. J Am Coll Cardiol 2002;39:202–9.

25. Nohria A, Tsang SW, Fang JC, et al. Clinical assessment identifies hemodynamic profiles that predict outcomes in patients admitted with heart failure. J Am Coll Cardiol 2003;41:1797–804.

26. Yancy CW, Jessup M, Bozkurt B, et al. 2013 ACCF/AHA guideline for the management of heart failure: a report of the American College of Cardiology Foundation/American Heart Association Task Force on Practice Guidelines. J Am Coll Cardiol 2013;62:e147–239.

27. Masip J, Peacock WF, Price S, et al. Indications and practical approach to non-invasive ventilation in acute heart failure. Eur Heart J 2018;39:17–25.

28. Thomas SS, Nohria A. Hemodynamic classifications of acute heart failure and their clinical application: an update. Circ J 2012;76:278–86.

29. Cohen MG, Kelly RV, Kong DF, et al. Pulmonary artery catheterization in acute coronary syndromes: insights from the GUSTO IIb and GUSTO III trials. Am J Med 2005;118:482–8.

30. Binanay C, Califf RM, Hasselblad V, et al. Evaluation study of congestive heart failure and pulmonary artery catheterization effectiveness: the ESCAPE trial. JAMA 2005;294:1625–33.

31. Swedberg K, Komajda M, Böhm M, et al. Ivabradine and outcomes in chronic heart failure (SHIFT): a randomised placebo-controlled study. Lancet 2010;376:875–85.

32. McMurray JJ, Packer M, Desai AS, et al. Angiotensin-neprilysin inhibition versus enalapril in heart failure. N Engl J Med 2014;371:993–1004.

33. Velazquez EJ, Morrow DA, DeVore AD, et al. Angiotensin-neprilysin inhibition in acute decompensated heart failure. N Engl J Med 2019;380:539–48.

34. McMurray JJV, Solomon SD, Inzucchi SE, et al. Dapagliflozin in patients with heart failure and reduced ejection fraction. N Engl J Med 2019;381:1995–2008.

35. Martinez FA, Serenelli M, Nicolau JC, et al. Efficacy and safety of dapagliflozin in heart failure with reduced ejection fraction according to age: insights from DAPA-HF. Circulation 2019. https://doi.org/10.1161/CIRCULATIONAHA.119.044133.

36. Marrouche NF, Brachmann J, Andresen D, et al. Catheter ablation for atrial fibrillation with heart failure. N Engl J Med 2018;378:417–27.

37. Di Biase L, Mohanty P, Mohanty S, et al. Ablation versus amiodarone for treatment of persistent atrial fibrillation in patients with congestive heart failure and an implanted device: results from the AATAC multicenter randomized trial. Circulation 2016;133:1637–44.

38. Berruezo A, Penela D, Jáuregui B, et al. Mortality and morbidity reduction after frequent premature ventricular complexes ablation in patients with left ventricular systolic dysfunction. Europace 2019;21:1079–87.

39. Velazquez EJ, Lee KL, Jones RH, et al. Coronary-artery bypass surgery in patients with ischemic cardiomyopathy. N Engl J Med 2016;374:1511–20.

40. Bertaina M, Galluzzo A, D'Ascenzo F, et al. Prognostic impact of MitraClip in patients with left ventricular dysfunction and functional mitral valve regurgitation: a comprehensive meta-analysis of RCTs and adjusted observational studies. Int J Cardiol 2019;290:70–6.

41. Maurer MS, Schwartz JH, Gundapaneni B, et al. Tafamidis treatment for patients with transthyretin amyloid cardiomyopathy. N Engl J Med 2018;379:1007–16.

42. SPRINT Research Group, Wright JT Jr, Williamson JD, Whelton PK, et al. A randomized trial of intensive versus standard blood-pressure control. N Engl J Med 2015;373:2103–16.

43. Jankowska EA, Tkaczyszyn M, Suchocki T, et al. Effects of intravenous iron therapy in iron-deficient patients with systolic heart failure: a meta-analysis of randomized controlled trials. Eur J Heart Fail 2016;18:786–95.

44. Blumenthal JA, Babyak MA, O'Connor C, et al. Effects of exercise training on depressive symptoms

in patients with chronic heart failure: the HF-ACTION randomized trial. JAMA 2012;308:465–74.

45. Reeves GR, Whellan DJ, O'Connor CM, et al. A novel rehabilitation intervention for older patients with acute decompensated heart failure: the REHAB-HF pilot study. JACC Heart Fail 2017;5: 359–66.

46. Metra M, Nodari S, D'Aloia A, et al. Beta-blocker therapy influences the hemodynamic response to inotropic agents in patients with heart failure: a randomized comparison of dobutamine and enoximone before and after chronic treatment with metoprolol or carvedilol. J Am Coll Cardiol 2002; 40:1248–58.

47. O'Connor CM, Gattis WA, Uretsky BF, et al. Continuous intravenous dobutamine is associated with an increased risk of death in patients with advanced heart failure: insights from the Flolan International Randomized Survival Trial (FIRST). Am Heart J 1999;138:78–86.

48. Lowes BD, Tsvetkova T, Eichhorn EJ, et al. Milrinone versus dobutamine in heart failure subjects treated chronically with carvedilol. Int J Cardiol 2001;81:141–9.

49. Cuffe MS, Califf RM, Adams KF Jr, et al. Short-term intravenous milrinone for acute exacerbation of chronic heart failure: a randomized controlled trial. JAMA 2002;287:1541–7.

50. Denton MD, Chertow GM, Brady HR. "Renal-dose" dopamine for the treatment of acute renal failure: scientific rationale, experimental studies and clinical trials. Kidney Int 1996;50:4–14.

51. Chen HH, Anstrom KJ, Givertz MM, et al. Low-dose dopamine or low-dose nesiritide in acute heart failure with renal dysfunction: the ROSE acute heart failure randomized trial. JAMA 2013;310:2533–43.

52. Stratton L, Berlin DA, Arbo JE. Vasopressors and Inotropes in Sepsis. Emerg Med Clin North Am 2017;35:75–91.

53. Hotchkiss Richard S, Lyle L. Sepsis and septic shock. Nat Rev Dis Primers 2016;2:16045.

54. Goldstein RE, Boccuzzi SJ, Cruess D, et al. Diltiazem increases late-onset congestive heart failure in postinfarction patients with early reduction in ejection fraction. The Adverse Experience Committee and the Multicenter Diltiazem Postinfarction Research Group. Circulation 1991;83:52–60.

55. Cotter G, Metzkor E, Kaluski E, et al. Randomised trial of high-dose isosorbide dinitrate plus low-dose furosemide versus high-dose furosemide plus low-dose isosorbide dinitrate in severe pulmonary oedema. Lancet 1998;351:389–93.

56. Matsue Y, Damman K, Voors AA, et al. Time-to-Furosemide treatment and mortality in patients hospitalized with acute heart failure. J Am Coll Cardiol 2017;69:3042–51.

57. Ellison DH. Diuretic therapy and resistance in congestive heart failure. Cardiology 2001;96:132–43.

58. Dormans TP, van Meyel JJ, Gerlag PG, et al. Diuretic efficacy of high dose furosemide in severe heart failure: bolus injection versus continuous infusion. J Am Coll Cardiol 1996;28:376–82.

59. Felker GM, Lee KL, Bull DA, et al. Diuretic strategies in patients with acute decompensated heart failure. N Engl J Med 2011;364:797–805.

60. Takei M, Kohsaka S, Shiraishi Y, et al. Effect of estimated plasma volume reduction on renal function for acute heart failure differs between patients with preserved and reduced ejection fraction. Circ Heart Fail 2015;8:527–32.

61. Trullàs JC, Morales-Rull JL, Casado J, et al. Rationale and design of the "safety and efficacy of the combination of loop with thiazide-type diuretics in patients with decompensated heart failure (CLOROTIC) trial:" a double-blind, randomized, placebo-controlled study to determine the effect of combined diuretic therapy (loop diuretics with thiazide-type diuretics) among patients with decompensated heart failure. J Card Fail 2016;22: 529–36.

62. De Vecchis R, Cantatrione C, Mazzei D, et al. The impact exerted on clinical outcomes of patients with chronic heart failure by aldosterone receptor antagonists: a meta-analysis of randomized controlled trials. J Clin Med Res 2017;9:130–42.

63. Gheorghiade M, Konstam MA, Burnett JC, et al. Short-term clinical effects of tolvaptan, an oral vasopressin antagonist, in patients hospitalized for heart failure: the EVEREST clinical status trials. JAMA 2007;297:1332–43.

64. Konstam MA, Gheorghiade M, Burnett JC, et al. Effects of oral tolvaptan in patients hospitalized for worsening heart failure: the EVEREST outcome trial. JAMA 2007;297:1319–31.

65. Konstam MA, Kiernan M, Chandler A, et al. Short-term effects of tolvaptan in patients with acute heart failure and volume overload. J Am Coll Cardiol 2017; 69:1409–19.

66. Felker GM, Mentz RJ, Cole RT, et al. Efficacy and safety of tolvaptan in patients hospitalized with acute heart failure. J Am Coll Cardiol 2017;69: 1399–406.

67. Thiele H, Zeymer U, Neumann FJ, et al. Intra-aortic balloon counterpulsation in acute myocardial infarction complicated by cardiogenic shock (IABP-SHOCK II): final 12 month results of a randomised, open-label trial. Lancet 2013;382:1638–45.

68. Thiele H, Zeymer U, Neumann FJ, et al. Intraaortic balloon support for myocardial infarction with cardiogenic shock. N Engl J Med 2012;367: 1287–96.

69. Nichol G, Karmy-Jones R, Salerno C, et al. Systematic review of percutaneous cardiopulmonary bypass for cardiac arrest or cardiogenic shock states. Resuscitation 2006;70:381–94.

70. Combes A, Leprince P, Luyt CE, et al. Outcomes and long-term quality-of-life of patients supported by extracorporeal membrane oxygenation for refractory cardiogenic shock. Crit Care Med 2008;36:1404–11.

71. Vallabhajosyula S, O'Horo JC, Antharam P, et al. Concomitant intra-aortic balloon pump use in cardiogenic shock requiring veno-arterial extracorporeal membrane oxygenation. Circ Cardiovasc Interv 2018;11:e006930.

72. Fincke R, Hochman JS, Lowe AM, et al. Cardiac power is the strongest hemodynamic correlate of mortality in cardiogenic shock: a report from the SHOCK trial registry. J Am Coll Cardiol 2004;44:340–8.

73. Burkhoff D, Cohen H, Brunckhorst C, et al. A randomized multicenter clinical study to evaluate the safety and efficacy of the TandemHeart percutaneous ventricular assist device versus conventional therapy with intraaortic balloon pumping for treatment of cardiogenic shock. Am Heart J 2006;152:469.e1-8.

74. Kar B, Gregoric ID, Basra SS, et al. The percutaneous ventricular assist device in severe refractory cardiogenic shock. J Am Coll Cardiol 2011;57:688–96.

75. Alkhouli M, Rihal CS, Holmes DR Jr. Transseptal techniques for emerging structural heart interventions. JACC Cardiovasc Interv 2016;9:2465–80.

76. Stevenson LW, Pagani FD, Young JB, et al. INTERMACS profiles of advanced heart failure: the current picture. J Heart Lung Transplant 2009;28:535–41.

Acute Decompensated Heart Failure in Patients with Heart Failure with Preserved Ejection Fraction

Tadafumi Sugimoto, MD, PhD, FESC

KEYWORDS

- Diagnosis • Exercise ventilation • Heart failure • Pulmonary circulation • Parathyroid hormone
- Right ventricular

KEY POINTS

- Right ventricular-to-pulmonary circulation coupling plays a crucial role in exercise ventilation in heart failure.
- Stepwise backward effects of loss in left atrial functional properties are a reduction in lung vessel compliance and vascular remodeling, which secondarily triggers right ventricular overload and dysfunction.
- Secondary hyperparathyroidism develops as a compensatory response to heart failure and contributes to calcium overload of the myocardium leading to cardiovascular disease.
- Prognostic impact of each parameter on acute decompensated heart failure patients is different at different points of time from admission to discharge.
- Exercise stress tests provide insight into the pathophysiology of heart failure, especially in the acute setting.

INTRODUCTION

Heart failure (HF) is a complex syndrome characterized by myocardial dysfunction, derangement of multiple organ systems, and poor outcome. Heart failure with preserved ejection fraction (HFpEF) comprises almost half of the population burden of HF. Even though there are several studies in diverse populations assessing the epidemiology of HFpEF, specific epidemiologic data on acute decompensated heart failure (ADHF) in HFpEF are currently lacking. An understanding of the disease process and the differences in clinical terms is necessary to manage ADHF patients correctly. In the patient management of ADHF with preserved ejection fraction (pEF), it is essential to know when and how to make a diagnosis and the right therapeutic decision. For this purpose, this review aims to summarize evidence of cause, diagnosis, and prognosis in both acute and chronic state of HFpEF and the exercise pathophysiology of HFpEF elucidating the potential pathophysiologic consequences of abnormal exercise response on the cardiovascular system in HFpEF.

Cause of Heart Failure with Preserved Ejection Fraction: Exercise Ventilation

Out of several markers of severity, abnormalities in exercise ventilation (VE) offer relevant insights into the pathophysiology of dyspnea, lung gas exchange, and control of ventilation and are recognized as substantial indicators of HF severity and

Department of Clinical Laboratory, Mie University Hospital, 2-174 Edobashi, Tsu 514-8507, Japan
E-mail address: t_sugimoto_japan@hotmail.com

Heart Failure Clin 16 (2020) 201–209
https://doi.org/10.1016/j.hfc.2019.12.002
1551-7136/20/© 2019 Elsevier Inc. All rights reserved.

prognosis.[1] An abnormal ventilatory response to exercise during an incremental workload is recognized as a hallmark manifestation of HF syndrome that reflects the mixed impairment of multiple organ systems and pathways and correlates with dyspnea sensation.[2] The origin of an increased and inefficient ventilatory response to exercise is multifactorial and primarily reflects how left ventricular (LV) dysfunction may impair lung physiology and both central and peripheral ventilatory control. The normal VE response to exercise implies a near-linear increase that is proportional to the progressive increase in carbon dioxide production (V_{CO_2}). For low and moderate intensity of work, this response is tightly regulated by arterial carbon dioxide partial pressure ($Paco_2$). At higher work intensities, the development of lactic acidosis and H^+ production from anaerobic prevailing metabolism further increases CO_2 release and the consequent amount of VE. An inefficient VE typically occurs in HF with either reduced ejection fraction [3–7] or pEF.[8,9] VE/V_{CO_2} slope, rather than their ratio, is generally endorsed by most laboratories and has been repeatedly identified as a strong and independent prognostic marker in different stages of heart disease.[3–7] Mathematically, the VE/V_{CO_2} slope is determined by 3 factors: the amount of CO_2 produced; the physiologic dead space/tidal volume ratio (VD/VT); and the $Paco_2$, and can be explained using the modified alveolar equation: $VE = 863 * V_{CO_2}/[Paco_2 * (1 - VD/VT)]$ (**Fig. 1**). Accordingly, the increased ventilator requirement in HF patients is determined by the behavior of arterial CO_2 tension during exercise and the fraction of the tidal volume going to the dead space. Three different mechanisms for an increased ventilatory requirement to a given CO_2 production have been reported in HF: (1) an increased waste ventilation, (2) early occurrence of decompensated acidosis, and (3) an abnormal chemoreflex and/or metaboreflex control.[10,11]

Several factors may explain an increased waste ventilation in HF patients, from either increased anatomic dead space (relative to low tidal volume)[12,13] or intrinsic pulmonary vascular changes and impaired vasoregulation[14,15] responsible for regional dishomogeneities in lung perfusion[16] and distribution of pulmonary blood flow.[17] In stable HF patients, a reduction in static lung mechanics (ie, reduced vital capacity and forced expiratory volume in 1 second)[12] is a common finding. The occurrence of restrictive lung changes is implicated in a lower rate of increase in tidal volume and higher respiratory rate and VD/VT for a given workload.[13] In agreement with an increased dead space ventilation role, there is also the demonstration that lung interstitial fibrosis and remodeling of alveolar-capillary membrane are additional features of changes occurring at the lung level in these patients.[18] Thus, occurrence of ventilation/perfusion mismatching and abnormalities in alveolar gas membrane conductance seem to be the pulmonary mediators of an uneven exercise VE in the increased ventilatory requirement during exercise. Recent studies have shown difference in pathophysiologic mechanisms underlying ventilatory efficiency during exercise between heart failure with reduced ejection fraction (HFrEF) and HFpEF.[19] Increasing VE/V_{CO_2} slope may be strongly explained by mechanisms influential in regulating $Paco_2$ in HFrEF, which contrasts with the strong role of increased VD/VT in HFpEF. Interestingly, in HFpEF patients at peak exercise, there is no difference in $Paco_2$ between younger and older patients, but dead space ventilation is greater in older compared with younger patients, suggesting a contribution to the processes of age-related exercise ventilatory inefficiency in HFpEF.[20] Additional hemodynamic factors, impaired right ventricular (RV) function and pulmonary hypertension that may generate some degree of RV to pulmonary circulation (PC) uncoupling, have been shown to play a crucial role in exercise capacity and ventilation in HF.[21–23]

Cause of Heart Failure with Preserved Ejection Fraction: Right Ventricular to Pulmonary Circulation Coupling and Left Atrial Function

Recent data have highlighted the growing importance of the right heart in clinical phenotyping and risk stratification in HFpEF.[24–29] RV dysfunction and pulmonary hypertension are common features in HFpEF, and both are powerful predictors of outcomes.[27–29] In HFpEF, the coupling of RV for a given overload pressure is commonly impaired,[23] so RV contractility gets worse with progressively higher vascular loading. Notably, RV-to-PC coupling has emerged as a comprehensive index of RV performance and right length-force relationship,[29] beyond the information provided per each variable in isolation.[23,30,31] Tricuspid plane annular systolic excursion (TAPSE) to pulmonary artery systolic pressure (PASP) ratio is a useful, simple, and noninvasive indicator of RV-PC coupling that has arisen in recent years.[30–33] On the other hand, the left atrium is extremely sensitive to sustained volume and pressure overload secondary to increased LV filling pressures,[34] and the stepwise backward effects of loss in left atrial (LA) functional properties are a reduction in lung vessel compliance and vascular remodeling that may trigger RV overload and dysfunction[35] (**Fig. 2**). In fact, the evolving stages

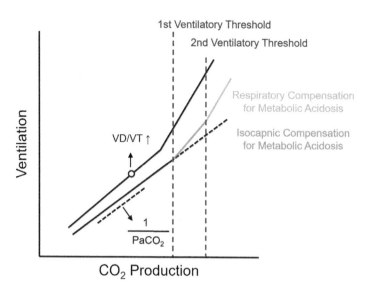

Fig. 1. Determinants of exercise ventilation. VD/VT, dead space to tidal volume ratio. Increased VD/VT causes an upward shift of the VE/V_{CO_2} slope.

of HFrEF or HFpEF are associated with RV-to-PC uncoupling, gas exchange impairment, and exercise ventilation inefficiency.[23,36] Before the development of a lung vascular remodeling process, the main determinant of an impaired right heart hemodynamic adaptation to exercise is the backward transmission of LA pressure, which is commonly caused by impeded LV filling, otherwise defined as increased pulsatile loading.[35] The LA remodeling in HFpEF and HFrEF differs, with greater eccentric LA remodeling in HFrEF and with increased stiffness, pulsatility, and predilection for atrial fibrillation in HFpEF.[37] An impaired LA reservoir function translates into a loss of pulmonary vessel compliance and has a strong hyperbolic correlation with the PASP/TAPSE ratio, a variable reflecting RV-to-PC coupling in both at rest and with exercise.[30,38,39] Moreover, exercise response of LA dynamics may be different between HFpEF and HFrEF, with an increase of LA reservoir function during exercise in HFpEF and without in HFrEF.[39]

Cause of Heart Failure with Preserved Ejection Fraction: Biomarker and Calcium-Parathyroid Hormone Axis

Recent study has reported in patients hospitalized with ADHF that HFpEF and HFrEF patients had higher levels of biomarkers related to inflammation and cardiac stretch, respectively, on admission, and biomarker levels of patients with HF with midrange ejection fraction (EF) were between HFrEF and HFpEF.[40] The origins of HF are rooted in inappropriate neurohormonal activation. Neurohormonal system includes the hypothalamic-pituitary-adrenal (HPA) axis, the adrenergic nervous system, and the renin-angiotensin-aldosterone system.[41,42] The activation of HPA axis with resultant release of adrenocorticotropin hormone promotes the adrenals' release of cortisol and aldosterone, and catecholamines from the adrenal medulla. The secondary aldosteronism of chronic HF contributes to increased fecal and urinary ionized calcium (Ca^{2+}) excretion

Fig. 2. RV-to-PC coupling and LA function. RAP, right atrial pressure; TRPG, tricuspid regurgitation peak gradient.

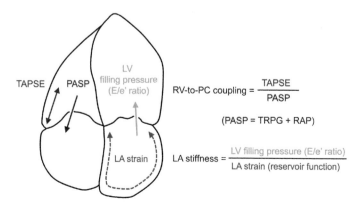

$$RV\text{-to-PC coupling} = \frac{TAPSE}{PASP}$$

$$(PASP = TRPG + RAP)$$

$$LA\ stiffness = \frac{LV\ filling\ pressure\ (E/e'\ ratio)}{LA\ strain\ (reservoir\ function)}$$

and consequent ionized hypocalcaemia and secondary hyperparathyroidism with elevated parathyroid hormone (PTH) levels.[43,44] The resulting increased PTH levels, in turn, stimulate synthesis of renin in juxta glomerular cells[45] and aldosterone in zona glomerulosa cells[46] by increasing intracellular Ca^{2+} levels. In addition, activation of the adrenergic nervous system with resultant elevated circulating catecholamines facilitates intracellular Ca^{2+} overloading with a subsequent decrease in plasma Ca^{2+}, which also provokes the parathyroid glands to release PTH,[47] potentially leading to secondary hyperparathyroidism. The parathyroid glands are 4 small oval bodies located on either side of the dorsal surface of the thyroid gland. PTH is secreted by the chief cells in the parathyroid gland, mainly in response to decreased circulating Ca^{2+} levels.[48] Changes in extracellular Ca^{2+} are sensed by the calcium-sensing receptors, which determine the response of the parathyroid to extracellular Ca^{2+} at the levels of PTH secretion, PTH gene expression, and parathyroid cell proliferation. The tight control of Ca^{2+} levels is essential for the maintenance of a plethora of processes, such as cell signaling, neuromuscular function, and bone metabolism. Recent studies showed the interrelationship between HF and PTH levels that PTH levels, even within the normal range, increase as pulmonary capillary wedge pressure (PCWP) increases and stroke volume decreases in patients with chronic HF.[49] Secondary hyperparathyroidism develops as a compensatory response to HF, but also contributes to Ca^{2+} overload of the myocardium, cardiac hypertrophy, and cardiac oxidative stress, leading to cardiovascular diseases (**Fig. 3**). In addition, PTH levels increase during exercise, resulting from decreasing circulating Ca^{2+} levels and metabolic acidosis.[50–52] Exercise-induced increase in PTH levels may have an acute catabolic effect on bone in no/low-impact activities (eg, cycling and cross-country skiing),[51] although high-impact activities (eg, volleyball) maintain or increase bone mineral density.

Diagnosis of Heart Failure with Preserved Ejection Fraction

LV diastolic dysfunction is attributed to age-related degeneration of heart and cardiovascular comorbidity potentially leading to HFpEF. Age-related changes in LV diastolic performance from normal to diastolic dysfunction are summarized that LV longitudinal strain (deformation) decreased with age, whereas LV circumferential and radial strain increased, and LA reservoir and conduit function decreased with age, whereas pump function increased, reflecting the age-related change in mitral inflow pattern[53,54] (**Fig. 4**). Recently, the American Society of Echocardiography/European Association of Cardiovascular Imaging recommended for assessment of LV diastolic function in patients with normal EF to evaluate 4 parameters: average E/e', septal/lateral e' velocity, tricuspid regurgitation

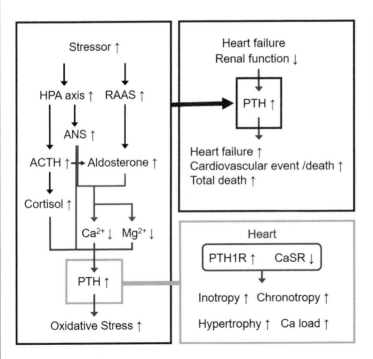

Fig. 3. Myocardial remodeling in HF with secondary hyperparathyroidism. ACTH, adrenocorticotropic hormone; ANS, autonomic nervous system; CaSR, calcium-sensing receptor; PTH1R, parathyroid hormone 1 receptor; RAAS, renin-angiotensin-aldosterone system.

	Gender	Age
Left Ventricular		
Longitudinal strain	♂ < ♀	↓
Circumferential strain	♂ < ♀	↑
Radial strain	♂ < ♀	↑
Left Atrial		
Reservoir function	♂ = ♀	↓
Pump function	♂ = ♀	↑
Conduit function	♂ = ♀	↓

Fig. 4. Sex differences and aging changes of the LV and LA strains in healthy subjects.

(TR) velocity, and LA volume index.[55] Because HFpEF can be defined by typical clinical symptoms (dyspnea, fatigue), normal left ventricular ejection fraction (LVEF; ≥50%), and elevated LV filling pressures (PCWP) at rest (>15 mm Hg) and/or with exercise (≥25 mm Hg),[23,56] diagnostic accuracy of echocardiography at rest and exercise for the diagnosis of HFpEF has been investigated. Obokata and colleagues[56] found that rest E/e' had high specificity and positive predictive value for HFpEF and, in contrast, exercise E/e' had high sensitivity and negative predictive value for HFpEF, although quantification of exercise PCWP was difficult by exercise E/e'. Belyavskiy and colleagues[57] reported the potential usefulness of diastolic stress testing using exercise E/e' and exercise TR velocity to diagnose HFpEF. Notably, most recent study has shown a close relationship between an impairment of LA functional property and elevated exercise PCWP accompanied by increased exercise pulmonary artery pressure, and significant HFpEF diagnostic utility of LA functional property.[58] In ADHF cohorts, LVEF were assessed at different points of time: on the admission day,[59] during the hospital stay,[60–63] and at follow-up visits after discharge.[64] Because of the hemodynamic difference in each point of time in ADHF, care should be taken when assessing LVEF. Indeed, recent study concerning the changes of LVEF in ADHF revealed that LVEF did not improve during hospitalization and improved after discharge in HFrEF; in contrast, LVEF improved during hospitalization in HFpEF without changes after discharge.[65]

Prognosis of Heart Failure with Preserved Ejection Fraction

Data from clinical studies on prognostic factors in HF patients are summarized in **Table 1**. Higher systolic blood pressure both at peak exercise and at admission for ADHF predicts better prognosis, reflecting LV contractile reserve, whereas higher systolic blood pressure at rest means higher risk in chronic HF. Oppositely, higher B-type natriuretic peptide (BNP) levels predict poor prognosis at rest and during the hospitalized period for ADHF both on admission and before discharge.[66] Regarding $Paco_2$, an inverse association was demonstrated between peak exercise $Paco_2$ and severity of HF, leading to poor prognosis. Importantly, in patients with acute HF irrespective of LVEF, one-third of patients have hypercapnia ($Paco_2$ at admission >45 mm Hg) characterized with HF symptom at rest, acute onset, and radiographic pulmonary edema, whereas one-third of patients have hypocapnia ($Paco_2$ <35 mm Hg).[63] The author's groups report interesting findings of diagnostic and prognostic impact of PTH levels in HF patients that PTH levels obtained in outpatients with HF were associated with the severity of HF and as an independent predictor of hospitalization for HF.[67] In the setting of chronic HF, Terrovitis and colleagues[68] have shown associations between increased PTH levels and decreased bone mineral density, leading to increased morbidity and mortality. In patients with ADHF, 60% of patients had an abnormal increase in PTH (>65 pg/mL) on admission, and low-normal PTH (10–40 pg/mL) was associated with increased all-cause mortality regardless of LVEF and renal function, suggesting that the compensatory response of PTH might contribute to cardiorenal protection.[69] On the other hand, Santas and colleagues[62] showed prognostic usefulness of the TAPSE/PASP ratio, as a noninvasive index of RV-to-PC coupling, in HFpEF patients discharged for acute HF. LA volume index and TR velocity were also reported as a prognostic factor in HFpEF patients with acute HF.[64] RV-to-PC coupling in ADHF might be attributed to LA functional reserve in HFpEF patients, similar to the relationship shown during exercise, although this needs to be verified. Actually, atrial fibrillation in patients with HFpEF predicts worse cardiovascular outcomes in those presenting with either an acute or a chronic presentation of HF, but not in those with HFrEF.[70,71]

Table 1
Prognostic factors in heart failure patients at different point of time

	Outpatient Clinic	During Exercise	On Admission	During Hospital Stay	Follow-Up Visits
HF					
Systolic blood pressure, mm Hg	Higher = Poor	Higher = Better	Higher = Better	—	Higher = Poor
Brain natriuretic peptide, pg/mL	Higher = Poor	—	Higher = Poor	Higher = Poor	Higher = Poor
$Paco_2$, mm Hg	—	Lower = Poor	Higher = Poor?	—	—
PTH, pg/mL	Higher = Poor	—	Higher = Better	—	Higher = Poor
HFpEF					
TAPSE/PASP, mm/mm Hg	Higher = Better	—	—	Higher = Better	—
LAVI, mL/m², and TR velocity, m/s	Higher = Poor	—	—	—	Higher = Poor

Abbreviation: LAVI, left atrial volume index.

Treatment of Acute Decompensated Heart Failure in Patients with Heart Failure with Preserved Ejection Fraction

ADHF is a life-threatening medical condition requiring urgent evaluation and treatment, typically leading to hospital admission.[72] In the urgent phase after the first medical contact of patients with suspected ADHF, patients should be assessed for cardiogenic shock and respiratory failure. Pharmacologic/mechanical circulatory support should be considered in cardiogenic shock with a diagnostic workup of acute HF. Ventilatory support (oxygen, noninvasive positive pressure ventilation, and mechanical ventilation) also should be considered in patients with respiratory failure, most typically patients with hypercapnia. In the immediate phase, the diagnosis of acute HF might be confirmed after excluding the presence of the following precipitants/causes leading to decompensation: acute coronary syndrome, hypertensive emergency, rapid arrhythmias or severe bradycardia/conduction disturbance, acute mechanical cause underlying acute HF, or acute pulmonary embolism. Nowadays there is no specific guideline-recommended treatment for ADHF in patients with HFpEF, but intravenous loop diuretics are recommended for all patients with acute HF admitted with signs/symptoms of fluid overload to improve symptoms.[72,73]

SUMMARY AND FUTURE DIRECTIONS

Cardiopulmonary exercise testing, invasive hemodynamic exercise testing, and exercise echocardiography are clearly useful in the assessment of HFpEF and provide detailed information to understand pathophysiology, define a specific phenotype, and elucidate the pathophysiologic consequences of impaired hemodynamic response and exercise ventilation inefficiency in HFpEF. There are only limited clinical studies concerning pathophysiology of ADHF in HFpEF, partially because of ununiformed diagnostic definition of HFpEF and different times of EF measurement in ADHF. More focused, well-designed studies are warranted to elucidate a potential association among gas exchange, hemodynamics, and calcium kinetics during exercise, which may have specific clinical implications targeting ADHF in patients with HFpEF.

DISCLOSURE

The author has nothing to disclose.

REFERENCES

1. Guazzi M. Abnormalities in cardiopulmonary exercise testing ventilatory parameters in heart failure: pathophysiology and clinical usefulness. Curr Heart Fail Rep 2014;11:80–7.

2. Arena R, Myers J, Guazzi M. The clinical and research applications of aerobic capacity and ventilatory efficiency in heart failure: an evidence-based review. Heart Fail Rev 2008;13(2):245–69.

3. Chua TP, Clark AL, Amadi AA, et al. Relation between chemosensitivity and the ventilatory response to exercise in chronic heart failure. J Am Coll Cardiol 1996;27:650–7.

4. Robbins M, Francis G, Pashkow FJ, et al. Ventilatory and heart rate responses to exercise–better predictors of heart failure mortality than peak oxygen consumption. Circulation 1999;100:2411–7.

5. Ponikowski P, Francis DP, Piepoli MF, et al. Enhanced ventilatory response to exercise in patients with chronic heart failure and preserved exercise tolerance–marker of abnormal cardiorespiratory reflex control and predictor of poor prognosis. Circulation 2001;103:967–72.

6. Guazzi M, Reina G, Tumminello G, et al. Exercise ventilation inefficiency and cardiovascular mortality in heart failure: the critical independent prognostic value of the arterial CO2 partial pressure. Eur Heart J 2005;26:472–80.

7. Arena R, Myers J, Abella J, et al. Development of a ventilatory classification system in patients with heart failure. Circulation 2007;115:2410–7.

8. Guazzi M, Myers J, Arena R. Cardiopulmonary exercise testing in the clinical and prognostic assessment of diastolic heart failure. J Am Coll Cardiol 2005;46:1883–90.

9. Maeder MT, Thompson BR, Htun N, et al. Hemodynamic determinants of the abnormal cardiopulmonary exercise response in heart failure with preserved left ventricular ejection fraction. J Card Fail 2012;18:702–10.

10. Ponikowski PP, Chua TP, Francis DP, et al. Muscle ergoreceptor overactivity reflects deterioration in clinical status and cardiorespiratory reflex control in chronic heart failure. Circulation 2001;104:2324–30.

11. Scott AC, Wensel R, Davos CH, et al. Skeletal muscle reflex in heart failure patients–role of hydrogen. Circulation 2003;107:300–6.

12. Wasserman K, Zhang YY, Gitt A, et al. Lung function and exercise gas exchange in chronic heart failure. Circulation 1997;96:2221–7.

13. Myers J, Salleh A, Buchanan N, et al. Ventilatory mechanisms of exercise intolerance in chronic heart failure. Am Heart J 1992;124:710–9.

14. Reindl I, Wernecke KD, Opitz C, et al. Impaired ventilatory efficiency in chronic heart failure: possible role of pulmonary vasoconstriction. Am Heart J 1998;136:778–85, 22.

15. Lewis GD, Shah RV, Pappagianopolas PP, et al. Determinants of ventilatory efficiency in heart failure: the role of right ventricular performance and pulmonary vascular tone. Circ Heart Fail 2008;1: 227–33.

16. Wada O, Asanoi H, Miyagi K, et al. Importance of abnormal lung perfusion in excessive exercise ventilation in chronic heart-failure. Am Heart J 1993;125: 790–8.

17. Wensel R, Georgiadou P, Francis DP, et al. Differential contribution of dead space ventilation and low arterial pCO(2) to exercise hyperpnea in patients with chronic heart-failure secondary to ischemic or idiopathic dilated cardiomyopathy. Am J Cardiol 2004;93:318–23.

18. Guazzi M, Reina G, Tumminello G, et al. Alveolar-capillary membrane conductance is the best pulmonary function correlate of exercise ventilation efficiency in heart failure patients. Eur J Heart Fail 2005;7:1017–22.

19. Van Iterson EH, Johnson BD, Borlaug BA, et al. Physiological dead space and arterial carbon dioxide contributions to exercise ventilatory inefficiency in patients with reduced or preserved ejection fraction heart failure. Eur J Heart Fail 2017;19:1675–85.

20. Smith JR, Borlaug BA, Olson TP. Exercise ventilatory efficiency in older and younger heart failure patients with preserved ejection fraction. J Card Fail 2019;25: 278–85.

21. Lewis GD, Murphy RM, Shah RV, et al. Pulmonary vascular response patterns during exercise in left ventricular systolic dysfunction predict exercise capacity and outcomes. Circ Heart Fail 2011;4: 276–85.

22. Guazzi M, Cahalin LP, Arena R. Cardiopulmonary exercise testing as a diagnostic tool for the detection of left-sided pulmonary hypertension in heart failure. J Card Fail 2013;19:461–7.

23. Borlaug BA, Kane GC, Melenovsky V, et al. Abnormal right ventricular-pulmonary artery coupling with exercise in heart failure with preserved ejection fraction. Eur Heart J 2016;37:3293–302.

24. Parikh KS, Sharma K, Fuizat M, et al. Heart failure with preserved ejection fraction expert panel report: current controversies and implications for clinical trials. JACC Heart Fail 2018;6:619–32.

25. Lewis SA, Schelbert EB, Williams SG, et al. Biological phenotypes of heart failure with preserved ejection fraction. J Am Coll Cardiol 2017;70:2186–200.

26. Santas E, Chorro FJ, Miñana G, et al. Tricuspid regurgitation and mortality risk across left ventricular systolic function in acute heart failure. Circ J 2015; 79:1526–33.

27. Gorter TM, Hoendermis ES, van Valdhuisen DJ, et al. Right ventricular dysfunction in heart failure with preserved ejection fraction: a systematic review and meta-analysis. Eur J Heart Fail 2016;18: 1472–87.

28. Lam CSP, Roger VL, Rodeheffer RJ, et al. Pulmonary hypertension in heart failure with preserved ejection fraction: a community-based study. J Am Coll Cardiol 2009;53:1119–26.

29. Guazzi M, Naeije M. Pulmonary hypertension in heart failure. J Am Coll Cardiol 2017;69:1718–34.

30. Guazzi M, Bandera F, Pelissero G, et al. Tricuspid annular plane systolic excursion and pulmonary arterial systolic pressure relationship in heart failure: an index of right ventricular contractile function and prognosis. Am J Physiol Heart Circ Physiol 2013; 305:1373–81.

31. Kaye DM, Marwick TH. Impaired right heart and pulmonary vascular function in HFpEF. Time for more risk markers? JACC Cardiovasc Imaging 2017;10: 1222–4.

32. Guazzi M, Dixon D, Labate V, et al. RV contractile function and its coupling to pulmonary circulation in heart failure with preserved ejection fraction: stratification of clinical phenotypes and outcomes. JACC Cardiovasc Imaging 2017;10:1211–21.

33. Gorter TM, van Veldhuisen DJ, Voors AA, et al. Right ventricular-vascular coupling in heart failure with preserved ejection fraction and pre- vs. post-capillary pulmonary hypertension. Eur Heart J Cardiovasc Imaging 2018;19:425–32.

34. Dernellis JM, Stefanadis CI, Zacharoulis AA, et al. Left atrial mechanical adaptation to long-standing hemodynamic loads based on pressure-volume relations. Am J Cardiol 1998;81:1138–43.

35. Guazzi M, Borlaug BA. Pulmonary hypertension due to left heart disease. Circulation 2012;126:975–90.

36. Guazzi M, Villani S, Generati G, et al. Right ventricular contractile reserve and pulmonary circulation uncoupling during exercise challenge in heart failure: pathophysiology and clinical phenotypes. JACC Heart Fail 2016;4:625–35.

37. Melenovsky V, Hwang SJ, Redfield MM, et al. Left atrial remodeling and function in advanced heart failure with preserved or reduced ejection fraction. Circ Heart Fail 2015;8:295–303.

38. Bandera F, Generati G, Pellegrino M, et al. Role of right ventricle and dynamic pulmonary hypertension on determining ΔVO2/Δwork rate flattening: insights from cardiopulmonary exercise test combined with exercise echocardiography. Circ Heart Fail 2014;7: 782–90.

39. Sugimoto T, Bandera F, Generati G, et al. Left atrial function dynamics during exercise in heart failure: pathophysiological implications on the right heart and exercise ventilation inefficiency. JACC Cardiovasc Imaging 2017;10:1253–64.

40. Tromp J, Khan MAF, Mentz RJ, et al. Biomarker profiles of acute heart failure patients with a mid-range ejection fraction. JACC Heart Fail 2017;5: 507–17.

41. Tan LB, Burniston JG, Clark WA, et al. Characterization of adrenoceptor involvement in skeletal and cardiac myotoxicity induced by sympathomimetic agents: toward a new bioassay for beta-blockers. J Cardiovasc Pharmacol 2003;41:518–25.

42. Benjamin IJ, Jalil JE, Tan LB, et al. Isoproterenol-induced myocardial fibrosis in relation to myocyte necrosis. Circ Res 1989;65:657–70.

43. Chhokar VS, Sun Y, Bhattacharya SK, et al. Hyperparathyroidism and the calcium paradox of aldosteronism. Circulation 2005;111:871–8.

44. Kamalov G, Deshmukh PA, Baburyan NY, et al. Coupled calcium and zinc dyshomeostasis and oxidative stress in cardiac myocytes and mitochondria of rats with chronic aldosteronism. J Cardiovasc Pharmacol 2009;53:414–23.

45. Saussine C, Judes C, Massfelder T, et al. Stimulatory action of parathyroid hormone on renin secretion in vitro: a study using isolated rat kidney, isolated rabbit glomeruli and superfused dispersed rat juxtaglomerular cells. Clin Sci (Lond) 1993;84:11–9.

46. Olgaard K, Lewin E, Bro S, et al. Enhancement of the stimulatory effect of calcium on aldosterone secretion by parathyroid hormone. Miner Electrolyte Metab 1994;20:309–14.

47. Borkowski BJ, Cheema Y, Shahbaz AU, et al. Cation dyshomeostasis and cardiomyocyte necrosis: the Fleckenstein hypothesis revisited. Eur Heart J 2011;32:1846–53.

48. Murray TM, Rao LG, Divieti P, et al. Parathyroid hormone secretion and action: evidence for discrete receptors for the carboxyl-terminal region and related biological actions of carboxyl-terminal ligands. Endocr Rev 2005;26:78–113.

49. Sugimoto T, Dohi K, Onishi K, et al. Interrelationship between haemodynamic state and serum intact parathyroid hormone levels in patients with chronic heart failure. Heart 2013;99:111–5.

50. Townsend R, Elliott-Sale KJ, Pinto AJ, et al. Parathyroid hormone secretion is controlled by both ionized calcium and phosphate during exercise and recovery in men. J Clin Endocrinol Metab 2016;101: 3231–9.

51. Kohrt WM, Wherry SJ, Wolfe P, et al. Maintenance of serum ionized calcium during exercise attenuates parathyroid hormone and bone resorption responses. J Bone Miner Res 2018;33:1326–34.

52. López I, Aguilera-Tejero E, Estepa JC, et al. Role of acidosis-induced increases in calcium on PTH secretion in acute metabolic and respiratory acidosis in the dog. Am J Physiol Endocrinol Metab 2004;286:E780–5.

53. Sugimoto T, Dulgheru R, Bernard A, et al. Echocardiographic reference ranges for normal left ventricular 2D strain: results from the EACVI NORRE study. Eur Heart J Cardiovasc Imaging 2017;18: 833–40.

54. Sugimoto T, Robinet S, Dulgheru R, et al. Echocardiographic reference ranges for normal left atrial function parameters: results from the EACVI NORRE study. Eur Heart J Cardiovasc Imaging 2018;19: 630–8.

55. Nagueh SF, Smiseth OA, Appleton CP, et al. Recommendations for the evaluation of left ventricular diastolic function by echocardiography: an update from the American Society of Echocardiography and the European Association of Cardiovascular Imaging. Eur Heart J Cardiovasc Imaging 2016;17: 1321–60.

56. Obokata M, Kane GC, Reddy YN, et al. Role of diastolic stress testing in the evaluation for heart failure with preserved ejection fraction: a simultaneous invasive-echocardiographic study. Circulation 2017;135:825–38.

57. Belyavskiy E, Morris DA, Url-Michitsch M, et al. Diastolic stress test echocardiography in patients with suspected heart failure with preserved ejection fraction: a pilot study. ESC Heart Fail 2019;6:146–53.

58. Telles F, Nanayakkara S, Evans S, et al. Impaired left atrial strain predicts abnormal exercise haemodynamics in heart failure with preserved ejection fraction. Eur J Heart Fail 2019;21:495–505.

59. Van Aelst LNL, Arrigo M, Placido R, et al. Acutely decompensated heart failure with preserved and reduced ejection fraction present with comparable haemodynamic congestion. Eur J Heart Fail 2018; 20:738–47.

60. Cho JH, Choe WS, Cho HJ, et al. Comparison of characteristics and 3-year outcomes in patients with acute heart failure with preserved, mid-range, and reduced ejection fraction. Circ J 2019;83: 347–56.

61. Yaku H, Ozasa N, Morimoto T, et al. Demographics, management, and in-hospital outcome of hospitalized acute heart failure syndrome patients in contemporary real clinical practice in Japan–observations from the prospective, multicenter Kyoto Congestive Heart Failure (KCHF) registry. Circ J 2018;82:2811–9.

62. Santas E, Palau P, Guazzi M, et al. Usefulness of right ventricular to pulmonary circulation coupling as an indicator of risk for recurrent admissions in heart failure with preserved ejection fraction. Am J Cardiol 2019;124(4):567–72.

63. Konishi M, Akiyama E, Suzuki H, et al. Hypercapnia in patients with acute heart failure. ESC Heart Fail 2015;2:12–9.

64. Donal E, Lund LH, Oger E, et al. Importance of combined left atrial size and estimated pulmonary pressure for clinical outcome in patients presenting with heart failure with preserved ejection fraction. Eur Heart J Cardiovasc Imaging 2017;18:629–35.

65. Yamamoto M, Seo Y, Ishizu T, et al. Different impact of changes in left ventricular ejection fraction between heart failure classifications in patients with acute decompensated heart failure. Circ J 2019; 83:584–94.

66. Hamatani Y, Nagai T, Shiraishi Y, et al. Long-term prognostic significance of plasma B-type natriuretic peptide level in patients with acute heart failure with reduced, mid-range, and preserved ejection fractions. Am J Cardiol 2018;121:731–8.

67. Sugimoto T, Tanigawa T, Onishi K, et al. Serum intact parathyroid hormone levels predict hospitalisation for heart failure. Heart 2009;95:395–8.

68. Terrovitis J, Zotos P, Kaldara E, et al. Bone mass loss in chronic heart failure is associated with secondary hyperparathyroidism and has prognostic significance. Eur J Heart Fail 2012;14:326–32.

69. Sugimoto T, Dohi K, Onishi K, et al. Prognostic value of serum parathyroid hormone level in acute decompensated heart failure. Circ J 2014;78:2704–10.

70. Go YY, Sugimoto T, Bulluck H, et al. Age and ejection fraction modify the impact of atrial fibrillation on acute heart failure outcomes. Eur J Heart Fail 2018;20:821–2.

71. Zafrir B, Lund LH, Laroche C, et al. Prognostic implications of atrial fibrillation in heart failure with reduced, mid-range, and preserved ejection fraction: a report from 14 964 patients in the European Society of Cardiology Heart Failure Long-Term Registry. Eur Heart J 2018;39:4277–84.

72. Ponikowski P, Voors AA, Anker SD, et al. 2016 ESC guidelines for the diagnosis and treatment of acute and chronic heart failure: the Task Force for the Diagnosis and Treatment of Acute and Chronic Heart Failure of the European Society of Cardiology (ESC) developed with the special contribution of the Heart Failure Association (HFA) of the ESC. Eur Heart J 2016;37:2129–200.

73. Yancy CW, Jessup M, Bozkurt B, et al. 2017 ACC/AHA/HFSA focused update of the 2013 ACCF/AHA guideline for the management of heart failure: a report of the American College of Cardiology/American Heart Association Task Force on Clinical Practice Guidelines and the Heart Failure Society of America. Circulation 2017;136:e137–61.

Acute Mitral Regurgitation and Transcatheter Mitral Valve Repair in an Emergency Case

Focus on the Mechanical Disorder of Mitral Valve Complex

Atsushi Hayashi, MD[a],*, Yogamaya Mantha, MD[b],
Rakushumimarika Harada, MD[b]

KEYWORDS

- Structure heart disease • Acute mitral regurgitation • MitraClip • Complication
- Mitral valve complex

KEY POINTS

- Acute mitral regurgitation has been a challenging disease that requires emergent care and proper management.
- Although echocardiography is essential for the diagnosis of acute mitral regurgitation, detection of an mitral regurgitation jet using color Doppler echocardiography is sometimes challenging owing to the acute elevation of left atrial pressure.
- In a patient with hemodynamic instability and high operative risk, a transcatheter mitral valve edge-to-edge repair using MitraClip system is a promising therapeutic option.

Acute mitral regurgitation (MR) is found infrequently, but is a challenging disease that requires emergent care and proper management.[1] Identifying the etiology and severity of MR are paramount to decision making. Moreover, it is essential to tailor management according to the severity of MR and subsequent hemodynamics compromise. Some of the uncommon cause of acute MR include sudden onset of leaflet tethering after acute myocardial infarction, transient systolic anterior motion of the mitral leaflet in the acute phase of Takotsubo cardiomyopathy, and penetrating or nonpenetrating chest trauma.[2–5] However, in this review article, we focus on the relatively common causes of acute primary MR from acute rupture of the chordae tendineae owing to myxomatous degeneration, iatrogenic complication, or infective endocarditis, and papillary muscle rupture after acute myocardial infarction.[6–9]

Acute MR is now receiving increased attention as one of the challenging areas in percutaneous mitral valve (MV) edge-to-edge repair using the MitraClip system (Abbott Vascular, Santa Clara, CA). Transcatheter MV repair has been well-established as a relatively safe treatment for patients with both chronic primary and secondary MR.[10–13] The feasibility of this procedure for acute MR has not been well-established, but some clinical cases reported that percutaneous MV repair for acute chordae rupture or papillary muscle rupture with

[a] Second Department of Internal Medicine, University of Occupational and Environmental Health, School of Medicine, Fukuoka, Japan; [b] Department of Internal Medicine, Texas Health Presbyterian Hospital of Dallas, 8200 Walnut Hill Lane, Dallas, TX, 75231, USA
* Corresponding author.
E-mail address: cherha524@med.uoeh-u.ac.jp

Heart Failure Clin 16 (2020) 211–219
https://doi.org/10.1016/j.hfc.2019.11.003
1551-7136/20/© 2019 Elsevier Inc. All rights reserved.

hemodynamic instability could be an effective treatment option for the patients who were at high risk for emergent surgical correction.[14,15]

CAUSES OF ACUTE MITRAL REGURGITATION

The MV is composed of the mitral annulus, mitral leaflets, and subvalvular apparatus, including the chordae tendineae and papillary muscles. The dysfunction or disruption of any parts of this MV complex can lead to acute MR. In general, spontaneous chordae rupture is the predominant cause of acute MR. Degenerative processes resulting in MR have 2 main phenotypes, myxomatous degeneration (so-called Barlow disease) and fibroelastic deficiency.[16–18] Patients with Barlow disease can have a genetic disorder and patients usually present in their fourth or fifth decade for symptomatic severe MR after a long history of regurgitation. In contrast, fibroelastic deficiency might be caused by an accelerated aging process and patients are typically older with more abrupt onset of MR; moderate or less MR in patients with fibroelastic deficiency can suddenly escalate to severe MR secondary to the rupture of weak chordae tendineae, leading to acute decompensated heart failure (**Fig. 1**).[16,17]

Infective endocarditis can affect both normal MV or preexisting degenerative MV.[19] Sudden onset chordae tendineae rupture owing to infective endocarditis in patients with relatively normal left ventricle and left atrium can cause a more severe hemodynamic instability than patients with preexisting degenerative MV who have a remodeled left ventricle and left atrium.

Papillary muscle rupture is a well-known mechanical complication of acute myocardial infarction, leading to acute MR with hemodynamic instability.[20,21] Severe MR usually occurs after a few days of right coronary artery occlusion without early revascularization. This is because the posteromedial papillary muscle has a single blood supply from the posterior descending branch of the right coronary artery, compared with the anterolateral papillary muscle, which receives blood from both the diagonal branch of the left anterior descending artery and the left circumflex artery.

Recently, chordae rupture associated with temporary left ventricular assist device implantations has been reported as the cause of acute MR.[7,22] The Impella (Abiomed, Danvers, MA) is a relatively new technology that has been used as a ventricular assist device to provide full circulatory support for patients presenting with cardiogenic shock.[23] Recent case report has shown that Impella device itself has potential to be caught at chordae tendinea, leading to chordae rupture and acute MR.[7]

DIAGNOSIS OF ACUTE MITRAL REGURGITATION

Owing to low cavity compliance in left atrium, a severe regurgitant volume can rapidly increase chamber pressure in left atrium to equalize pressure between left atrium and left ventricle, which cause a rapid decrease in regurgitant volume during mid to late systole. That is why the auscultatory finding with a soft systolic murmur that diminishes or disappears in mid to late systole may make you misunderstand the severity of MR.

Echocardiography plays an essential role in the diagnosis of acute primary MR.[24] However, acute severe MR is more challenging to diagnose than chronic severe MR using transthoracic echocardiography.[1,25] The normal left atrium and left ventricular size with hypercontraction of the left ventricle may be misleading. Further, color Doppler imaging in acute MR frequently will not show a large turbulent flow disturbance owing to the acute increase in left atrial pressure with low blood pressure, and thus MR may be underestimated or not appreciated at all. Thus, a comprehensive approach is required. The abnormal signs of the MV complex, such as ruptured chordae, flail leaflets, and complete ruptured papillary muscle with normal size of left atrium and left ventricle, help to make a diagnosis of severe acute MR. Incomplete or impending papillary muscle rupture secondary to acute myocardial infarction can cause severe acute MR, but it is not easy to find these papillary muscle abnormalities. In this setting, regional wall motion abnormalities of the left ventricle underlying the papillary muscle in addition to the MV prolapse with relatively normal leaflet characteristics (thickness or length) is the important sign suggesting the severe MR. An early peaking or cutoff sign by continuous Doppler echocardiography represents the acute increase in left atrial pressure and is particularly informative in this setting (see **Fig. 1**C). The flow reversal in the pulmonary veins may help support the diagnosis of severe MR but may not be reliable in the setting of tachycardia and atrial fibrillation. In contrast, quantification of regurgitant volume or effective regurgitant orifice area, which are usually recommended in the evaluation of the severity of chronic MR,[26] is often difficult in patients with acute MR and congestive heart failure because of rapid heart rate or fast breathing rate. Accordingly, transesophageal echocardiography (TEE) is encouraged for a more definite diagnosis and improved patients' management.

When placing transcatheter devices, such as a transcatheter aortic valve or microaxial rotary blood pump, a pigtail catheter, curved guidewire,

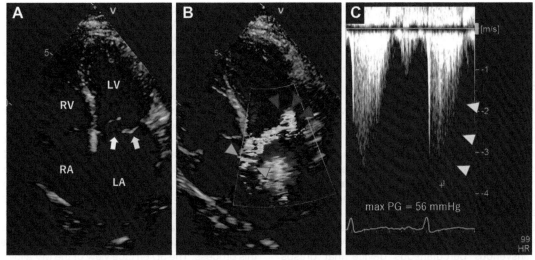

Fig. 1. A case of acute MR. (*A*) Transthoracic echocardiography image of the four-chamber view showing flail P2+P3 segment (*yellow arrow*). The ruptured chordae can be clearly visualized (*white arrow*). (*B*) Color flow image showing an acceleration flow signal (*red arrowhead*) and antero-medial directed wall jet (*green arrowhead*). Jet area in the left atrium is relatively small in spite of a huge acceleration flow signal area. (*C*) The continuous wave Doppler recording of the MR velocity showing cut-off sign, which demonstrates an acute increase in the left atrium pressure. LA, left atrium; LV, left ventricle; PG, pressure gradient; RA, right atrium; RV, right ventricle.

or the device in the left ventricle can unexpectedly hook the chordae.[6,7] A careful guidance and evaluation with transthoracic echocardiography or TEE becomes critical in avoiding irreversible MV or subvalvular damage. An acute increase in pulmonary artery wedge pressure or acute decrease in systemic blood pressure may be a sign of development of acute MR. If the ruptured chordae with a flail MV leaflet is unfortunately observed, emergent surgical MV repair should be considered.

MANAGEMENT OF ACUTE MITRAL REGURGITATION

There are various treatment options for patients with acute MR, which should be selected based on the hemodynamic status, etiologies of valve dysfunction, and other comorbidities.[26,27] Vasodilator therapy can be useful to improve hemodynamic compensation seen in patients with moderate or less acute MR by decreasing the impedance of aortic flow and increasing the forward output. However, medical therapies have a limited role in acute severe MR; thus, intra-aortic balloon counterpulsation should be considered to decreases afterload and increases aortic diastolic pressure. The intra-aortic balloon pump can be used as a temporary cardiac support until patients undergo surgical repair. Additionally, left ventricular assist device such as Impella Recover device or venoarterial extracorporeal membrane oxygenation

can also be used to improve cardiac output and oxygenation in patients with cardiogenic shock.[28]

Acute MR is associated with worse short-term outcome.[29] Accordingly, emergent surgical correction is usually required. In patients with decompensated heart failure caused by acute severe MR from spontaneous, iatrogenic, or myxomatous ruptured chordae tendineae, an urgent MV repair is recommended in preference to MV replacement, as with the chronic primary MR. In patients with infective endocarditis, the optimal timing of intervention is unclear, but early surgical intervention is strongly indicated for patients with decompensated heart failure secondary to mitral valvular vegetation or annular abscess.[30] A rupture of a papillary muscle as a complication from acute myocardial infarction also requires an urgent surgical correction.[8,20] When a partial papillary muscle rupture without a hemodynamic compromise is observed, it requires an urgent surgery because it can suddenly progress to complete papillary muscle rupture. Although MV replacement is generally performed, some case reports have shown that MV repair is a feasible treatment option for acute papillary muscle rupture with improved mortality and long-term outcomes.[31,32]

A few case reports have demonstrated an improved outcome with percutaneous MV repair using MitraClip system for patients with higher operative risks presenting with acute MR from ruptured papillary muscles or tendons.[21,33,34] Although it is an off-label use of the MitraClip, percutaneous repair is a promising therapeutic option alternative to surgical correction for such patients with prohibitive risk for surgery.

PERCUTANEOUS TRANSCATHETER INTERVENTION AND THE ROLE OF ECHOCARDIOGRAPHY

In the last decades, percutaneous MV repair of primary chronic MR has successfully treated patients who are considered high risk for surgical valve intervention. The percutaneous approach is completed by a procedure that creates a double orifice valve and reestablishes leaflet coaptation, approximating the distance between the anterior and posterior mitral leaflet edges.[10,11] This leaflet plication technology is based on the surgical Alfieri technique.[35] The MitraClip, a transvenous percutaneous device that grasps both anterior and posterior MV leaflets and thereby reduces MR, was first performed in patients in 2003.[36] It received CE mark approval in 2008 and approval from the US Food and Drug Administration in 2013 specifically for primary or degenerative lesions.

The MitraClip system consists of the clip delivery system, a device that is mounted at its distal end, and a steerable guide catheter (**Fig. 2**). The MitraClip comes in 2 sizes (NTR/XTR) and it is made of cobalt chromium metal alloy covered by poly-propylene fabric. The steerable guide catheter is 24F proximally, and tapers to 22F when it gains access to the left atrium at the level of the atrial septum through a transseptal puncture. The clip arms of NTR is 9 mm long and XTR has its arm of 12 mm. The width of 2 arms in opened position are approximately 2 cm in NTR and 2.5 cm in XTR. The width of the clips itself is 4 mm in NTR and 5 mm in XTR.

The procedure is performed under general anesthesia with the use of fluoroscopic and 2-dimensional (2D) and 3-dimensional (3D) TEE guidance. Especially, TEE imaging is integral to the procedure success. Its role in assessing suitability for the treatment, procedural guidance, and evaluating results of clipping has been reviewed in detail previously.[37] In this paragraph, an appreciation for the key points and potential pitfalls of each step during percutaneous edge-to-edge repair for acute MR was briefly reviewed.

The transseptal puncture is the first step. Using a modified mid-esophageal aortic short axis view and the orthogonal view that displays superior, inferior, anterior, and posterior rims of the interatrial septum, the transseptal sheath/needle should be positioned posteriorly with the height of 4 to 5 cm above the plane of the mitral annulus or leaflet coaptation (**Fig. 3**A–C). In patients with acute MR, a small left atrium may limit a position of the septal puncture enough to the height from the mitral annulus, that, after the puncture, the steerable guide catheter is advanced until approximately 2 cm of the catheter is across the septum under continuous 2D and 3D TEE guidance. Wide sector full-volume live 3D imaging is useful to visualize the catheter and its relationship with other structures. The clip delivery system is advanced beyond the steerable guide catheter into the left atrium under wide sector full-volume 3D TEE or 2D TEE guidance (**Fig. 4**). Careful adjustment of the scan plane angle to elongate the entire clip system is needed to avoid the left atrial injury. Patients with a small left atrium have increased risks of left atrial perforation by clip delivery system at this process. The 3D en face view of the MV allows for orientation of the clip graspers aligned above the origin of the MR jet and the clip is opened to extend the 2 arms (see **Fig. 4**B). The clip is advanced into the left ventricle below the mitral leaflets and appropriately positioned in the left ventricle under 2D TEE simultaneous orthogonal midcommissural and long axis views guidance (see **Fig. 4**C). Once appropriately positioned in the left ventricle, the expanded clip is slowly withdrawn slightly, allowing the leaflets to fall into the arms. Simultaneous orthogonal biplane 2D TEE imaging help grasp the leaflet edges by the clip arms (**Fig. 5**). A successful grasping results in immediate reduction in the MR flow. An assessment of leaflet insertion is made to ensure the stability of the device and leaflets from 2D TEE midesophageal left ventricular long axis view (see **Fig. 5**C). Leaflet capture can be challenging in patients with a significant coaptation defect, for example, in patients with a large flail gap. If adequate MR reduction is observed by 2D and 3D TEE color Doppler images, the clip is released. Importantly, although cumulative vena contracta areas by 3D TEE color Doppler echocardiography may allow for accurate quantitative method for assessment of MR severity, there are many limitations in this method, for example, temporal resolution, special resolution, and various artifacts (see **Fig. 5**D).[38–40] In clinical settings, a comprehensive approach, including 2D color Doppler MR jet areas, mean transmitral gradient, and pulmonary venous flow velocity, is useful to evaluate the results of clipping.[41,42] It is important to ensure that hemodynamic condition during the MitraClip procedure for acute MR is tremendously varied from the postprocedural condition. The second clip is considered if the degree of MR reduction from the first clip is insufficient and mitral stenosis is not significant.

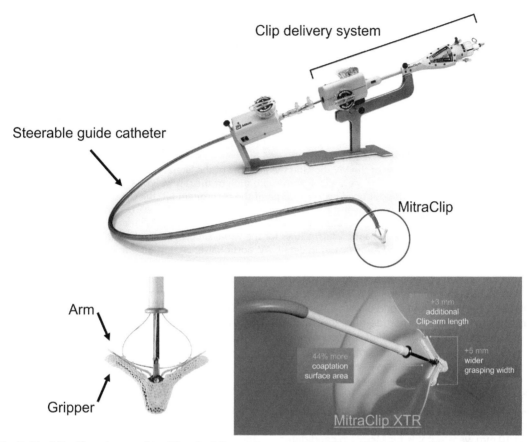

Fig. 2. The MitraClip system consists of the clip delivery system and a steerable guide catheter. A clip, consisting of an arm and a gripper, is attached to the tip of the delivery system. The MitraClip XTR, the third generation of MitraClip, has longer clip arms and wider grippers, which is expected to treat more complex cases with easier grasping and better reach. (Mitra-Clip is a trademark of Abbott or its related companies. Reproduced with permission of Abbott, © 2019. All rights reserved.)

FAVORABLE VALVE ANATOMY FOR THE MitraClip

In addition to the clinical selection criteria based on the valvular heart disease guidelines,[30] a careful evaluation of the MV morphology by echocardiography is also required to look for optimal candidate for undergoing the MitraClip placements.[37] The EVEREST trials, the initial gold standard for selection criteria for MitraClip, include

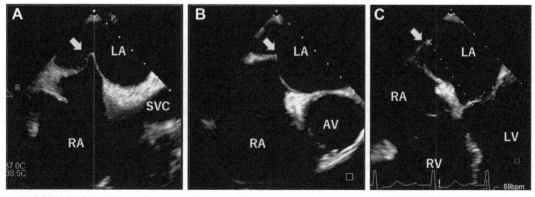

Fig. 3. (A) 2D TEE bicaval view of the interatrial septum (IAS) showing the transseptal needle tenting the IAS (*yellow arrow*). (B) The needle posteriorly positioned is identified using aortic short axis view. On this view, aortic valve serves as an anterior reference point. (C) The distance from the intended septal puncture point to the annular plane is measured using the modified 4-chamber view. AV, aortic valve; LA, left atrium; LV, left ventricle; RA, right atrium; RV, right ventricle; SVC, superior vena cava.

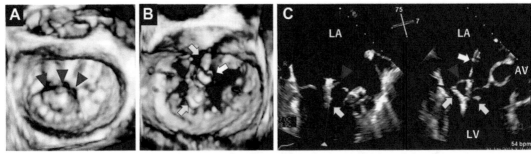

Fig. 4. (*A*) A 3D TEE en face view of the MV showing the prolapse of the lateral site of P2 scallop (*red arrowheads*). (*B*) Visualization of MV in 3D en face view allows for visualization of the clip (*yellow arrows*) in relation to the line of coaptation. Once the clip is positioned over the origin of the regurgitant jet, the clip delivery system (*white arrow*) is advanced into the left ventricle just below the mitral leaflet edges. (*C*) A 2D TEE simultaneous orthogonal midcommissural and long-axis views. Simultaneous multiplane imaging permits the use of a dual screen to simultaneously display 2 real-time 2D images, which allows for the visualization of the relationships between clip arms (*yellow arrows*) and leaflets (*red arrowheads*) in detail. AV, aortic valve; LA, left atrium; LV, left ventricle.

only limited patients with favorable valve anatomy to achieve optimal outcomes and, therefore, do not reflect the clinical real world of MitraClip candidates. For example, a chordae-free zone in the central part of the anterior leaflet was considered more suitable for the clipping compared with the medial and lateral segments, where the complex structure of the chordae tendineae is attached, which might increase the risk of clip entanglement.[43] Furthermore, patients with flail segment widths of less than 15 mm and flail gaps of less than 10 mm were suitable for MitraClip candidates to achieve its feasibility, safety, and effectiveness.[10,44] With the increasing use of and experience with the MitraClip, the results of recent studies and registries challenged the concept that MV anatomy beyond the EVEREST trials could be associated with worse clinical outcomes.

Estevez-Loureiro and colleagues[43] focused on the noncentral MV prolapse, which included both medial and lateral regions of the mitral leaflets. In this study where MitraClip placements were performed by experienced physicians, a percutaneous edge-to-edge repair was feasible to treat the noncentral MR with significant reduction of MR, left ventricle size, and clinical events. Attizzani and colleagues[45] showed that extended use of percutaneous edge-to-edge repair beyond EVEREST criteria was acceptable with similar rates of safety and efficacy through 12-month follow-up compared with control subjects who were fulfilled with the EVEREST criteria. Other study showed that there was no difference between the Efficacy and Failure group according to the adherence of EVEREST criteria.[46] Additionally, there comes a new-generation MitraClip system, the MitraClip XTR system, which may facilitate percutaneous edge-to-edge repair particularly in complex cases, or even make previously unpromising cases possible.[47] Given that only

experience centers with percutaneous MV repair can attempt to treat patients who are not meet EVEREST criteria, more patients with acute MR and high risks for surgical MV correction can be treated by percutaneous catheter intervention.

MitraClip FOR ACUTE MITRAL REGURGITATION

Patients with acute primary MR who are not eligible for conventional MV surgery could have the therapeutic option of transcatheter management. Off-label use of MitraClip is the only clinically available method in this patient population.

Most studies investigating the safety and effectiveness of the MitraClip for severe MR excluded patients with acute MR. Thus, limited evidence is available on emergency MitraClip therapy for the management of acute MR and cardiogenic shock. Adamo and colleagues[33] reported single-center experience in 5 consecutive patients admitted owing to acute MI complicated by severe MR associated with severe hemodynamic impairment. All patients had severe MR that developed after successful emergency percutaneous coronary intervention. Hemodynamic instability persisted with an inability to wean patients from mechanical support and intravenous drugs. All patients underwent successful urgent implantation of the MitraClip with significant improvement of cardiogenic shock. Valle and colleagues[21] reported a single case of a 84-year-old man with inferoposterior ST elevation myocardial infarction and MR4+ with a partial tear of the papillary muscle. After complete revascularization, hemodynamic instability persisted; therefore, patient was successfully treated with MitraClip, deploying 3 clips and producing a single residual lateral orifice, with a favorable outcome at 6 weeks.

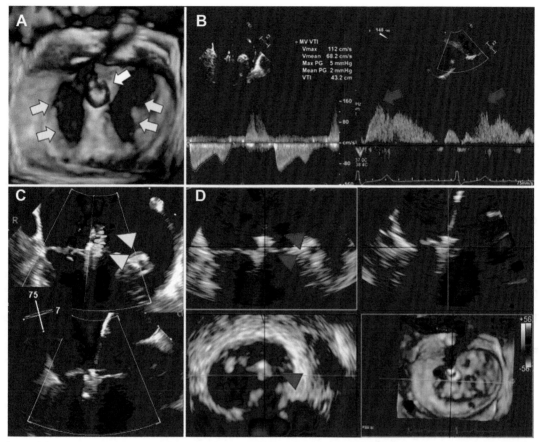

Fig. 5. (*A*) A 3D TEE en face view of the MV showing the placement of the clip (*white arrow*) resulting in a double orifice valve (*yellow arrows*). (*B*) The assessment of the residual significant MR and stenosis is performed using the continuous wave Doppler recording across one of the double orifices of the MV and the change in systolic flow velocity of pulmonary vein flow before and after the clipping. Mean mitral diastolic gradient should be less than 5 mm Hg (*left side* of *B*). Systolic wave of pulmonary vein flow in patients with severe MR is usually reversal and negative. However, systolic wave of pulmonary vein flow increases from negative to positive after the clipping (*red arrows*), which represents a decrease in MR and left atrial pressure (*right side* of *B*). (*C, D*) The degree of residual MR was evaluated using 2D and 3D TEE color Doppler imaging. There was mild MR after clipping in the 2D TEE image in the midcommissural view (*yellow arrowheads*). However, it was sometimes difficult to quantitate MR by vena contracta area using cross-sectional cut plane of the 3D TEE color Doppler image (*red arrowheads*). This is because of the lower temporal and special resolution of 3D color Doppler image compared with these of 2D image. To overcome these limitations, focus only on the regurgitant orifice and minimize the sector width and depth.

There are some particular difficulties associated with the emergence of percutaneous interventions for acute valvular diseases unlike the elective intervention for chronic valvular diseases. Specifically, in addition to the serious patients' condition with cardiogenic shock and pulmonary edema, relatively small left atrium may not allow to get adequate image quality of the TEE during the percutaneous procedure. Furthermore, a small left atrium could make it difficult to approach appropriate or accurate transseptal puncture, which may add complexity to the procedure or result in iatrogenic injury. Small left ventricle may also make the procedure more difficult because

the chordae tendineae in the small cavity can prevent the clip from grasping leaflets safely. In addition, patients with acute papillary muscle rupture after myocardial infarction have prominent mitral bileaflet prolapse, which may increase the chance for the procedural failure. Further studies evaluating the role of transcatheter approaches for management of acute MR are needed.

SUMMARY

The diagnosis of acute MR is often missed or delayed because the clinical presentation is substantially different from that in patients with chronic MR. Management of acute MR depends on the specific etiology of valve dysfunction. Echocardiography has been central to the diagnosis of acute MR. High mortality remains as the main problem, despite improvement in surgical intervention and revascularization strategies. To avoid catastrophic consequences, percutaneous MV edge-to-edge repair using MitraClip may have a key role in the treatment of unstable patients with acute primary MR who are at high surgical risks. Further experience and evidence are required to make this therapy more standard therapy for acute MR.

ACKNOWLEDGMENTS

The authors thank Kazuma Nagayoshi, from Abbott Vascular Japan, for his assistance.

DISCLOSURE

The authors have nothing to disclose.

REFERENCE

1. Zipes D, Bonow RO, Mann DL, et al. Braunwald's heart disease: a textbook of cardiovascular medicine. 11th edition. Philadelphia: Elsevier; 2019.
2. Nishino S, Watanabe N, Kimura T, et al. Acute versus chronic ischemic mitral regurgitation: an echocardiographic study of anatomy and physiology. Circ Cardiovasc Imaging 2018;11(4):e007028.
3. Izumo M, Nalawadi S, Shiota M, et al. Mechanisms of acute mitral regurgitation in patients with takotsubo cardiomyopathy: an echocardiographic study. Circ Cardiovasc Imaging 2011;4(4):392–8.
4. Bouabdallaoui N, Wang Z, Lecomte M, et al. Acute mitral regurgitation in Takotsubo cardiomyopathy. Eur Heart J Acute Cardiovasc Care 2015;4(2): 197–9.
5. Elapavaluru S, Alhassan S, Khan F, et al. Severe acute traumatic mitral regurgitation, cardiogenic shock secondary to embolized polymethylmethracrylate cement foreign body after a percutaneous vertebroplasty. Ann Thorac Surg 2016;101(3): 1169–71.
6. Joseph M, Perry R, Sinhal A, et al. Acute mitral regurgitation complicating transcatheter aortic valve implantation. J Heart Valve Dis 2011;20(3):361–3.
7. Elhussein TA, Hutchison SJ. Acute mitral regurgitation: unforeseen new complication of the Impella LP 5.0 ventricular assist device and review of literature. Heart Lung Circ 2014;23(3):e100–4.
8. Austen WG, Sokol DM, DeSanctis RW, et al. Surgical treatment of papillary-muscle rupture complicating myocardial infarction. N Engl J Med 1968;278(21): 1137–41.
9. Nishimura RA, Schaff HV, Shub C, et al. Papillary muscle rupture complicating acute myocardial infarction: analysis of 17 patients. Am J Cardiol 1983;51(3):373–7.
10. Feldman T, Wasserman HS, Herrmann HC, et al. Percutaneous mitral valve repair using the edge-to-edge technique: six-month results of the EVEREST phase I clinical trial. J Am Coll Cardiol 2005; 46(11):2134–40.
11. Feldman T, Kar S, Rinaldi M, et al. Percutaneous mitral repair with the MitraClip system: safety and midterm durability in the initial EVEREST (Endovascular Valve Edge-to-Edge REpair Study) cohort. J Am Coll Cardiol 2009;54(8):686–94.
12. Feldman T, Foster E, Glower DD, et al. Percutaneous repair or surgery for mitral regurgitation. N Engl J Med 2011;364(15):1395–406.
13. Maisano F, Franzen O, Baldus S, et al. Percutaneous mitral valve interventions in the real world: early and 1-year results from the ACCESS-EU, a prospective, multicenter, nonrandomized post-approval study of the MitraClip therapy in Europe. J Am Coll Cardiol 2013;62(12):1052–61.
14. Estevez-Loureiro R, Arzamendi D, Freixa X, et al. Percutaneous mitral valve repair for acute mitral regurgitation after an acute myocardial infarction. J Am Coll Cardiol 2015;66(1):91–2.
15. Papadopoulos K, Chrissoheris M, Nikolaou I, et al. Edge-to-edge mitral valve repair for acute mitral valve regurgitation due to papillary muscle rupture: a case report. Eur Heart J Case Rep 2019;3(1): ytz001.
16. Anyanwu AC, Adams DH. Etiologic classification of degenerative mitral valve disease: Barlow's disease and fibroelastic deficiency. Semin Thorac Cardiovasc Surg 2007;19(2):90–6.
17. Adams DH, Rosenhek R, Falk V. Degenerative mitral valve regurgitation: best practice revolution. Eur Heart J 2010;31(16):1958–66.
18. Chandra S, Salgo IS, Sugeng L, et al. Characterization of degenerative mitral valve disease using morphologic analysis of real-time three-dimensional echocardiographic images: objective insight into complexity and planning of mitral valve repair. Circ Cardiovasc Imaging 2011;4(1):24–32.
19. Hoen B, Duval X. Infective endocarditis. N Engl J Med 2013;369(8):785.
20. Thompson CR, Buller CE, Sleeper LA, et al. Cardiogenic shock due to acute severe mitral regurgitation complicating acute myocardial infarction: a report from the SHOCK trial registry. SHould we use emergently revascularize Occluded Coronaries in cardiogenic shocK? J Am Coll Cardiol 2000;36(3 Suppl A): 1104–9.
21. Valle JA, Miyasaka RL, Carroll JD. Acute mitral regurgitation secondary to papillary muscle tear: is transcatheter edge-to-edge mitral valve repair a

new paradigm? Circ Cardiovasc Interv 2017;10(6) [pii:e005050].

22. Bhatia N, Richardson TD, Coffin ST, et al. Acute mitral regurgitation after removal of an Impella device. Am J Cardiol 2017;119(8):1290–1.

23. Han JJ, Acker MA, Atluri P. Left ventricular assist devices. Circulation 2018;138(24):2841–51.

24. Goldman AP, Glover MU, Mick W, et al. Role of echocardiography/Doppler in cardiogenic shock: silent mitral regurgitation. Ann Thorac Surg 1991;52(2): 296–9.

25. Watanabe N. Acute mitral regurgitation. Heart 2019; 105(9):671–7.

26. Nishimura RA, Otto CM, Bonow RO, et al. 2014 AHA/ ACC guideline for the management of patients with valvular heart disease: executive summary: a report of the American College of Cardiology/American Heart Association Task Force on practice guidelines. J Am Coll Cardiol 2014;63(22):2438–88.

27. Baumgartner H, Falk V, Bax JJ, et al. 2017 ESC/ EACTS guidelines for the management of valvular heart disease. Eur Heart J 2017;38(36):2739–91.

28. Foerst J, Cardenas A, Swank G. Safety of MitraClip implant in the unstable patient: feasibility of concomitant left ventricular support device. JACC Cardiovasc Interv 2016;9(7):e71–2.

29. Tcheng JE, Jackman JD Jr, Nelson CL, et al. Outcome of patients sustaining acute ischemic mitral regurgitation during myocardial infarction. Ann Intern Med 1992;117(1):18–24.

30. Nishimura RA, Otto CM, Bonow RO, et al. 2014 AHA/ ACC guideline for the management of patients with valvular heart disease: a report of the American College of Cardiology/American Heart Association Task Force on practice guidelines. J Am Coll Cardiol 2014;63(22):e57–185.

31. Fasol R, Lakew F, Wetter S. Mitral repair in patients with a ruptured papillary muscle. Am Heart J 2000; 139(3):549–54.

32. Sultan I, Aranda-Michel E, Gleason TG, et al. Mitral valve surgery for acute papillary muscle rupture. J Card Surg 2018;33(9):484–8.

33. Adamo M, Curello S, Chiari E, et al. Percutaneous edge-to-edge mitral valve repair for the treatment of acute mitral regurgitation complicating myocardial infarction: a single centre experience. Int J Cardiol 2017;234:53–7.

34. Alkhouli M, Wolfe S, Alqahtani F, et al. The feasibility of transcatheter edge-to-edge repair in the management of acute severe ischemic mitral regurgitation. JACC Cardiovasc Interv 2017;10(5):529–31.

35. Maisano F, Torracca L, Oppizzi M, et al. The edge-to-edge technique: a simplified method to correct mitral insufficiency. Eur J Cardiothorac Surg 1998; 13(3):240–5 [discussion: 245–6].

36. St Goar FG, Fann JI, Komtebedde J, et al. Endovascular edge-to-edge mitral valve repair: short-term results in a porcine model. Circulation 2003;108(16):1990–3.

37. Nyman CB, Mackensen GB, Jelacic S, et al. Transcatheter mitral valve repair using the edge-to-edge clip. J Am Soc Echocardiogr 2018;31(4):434–53.

38. Altiok E, Hamada S, Brehmer K, et al. Analysis of procedural effects of percutaneous edge-to-edge mitral valve repair by 2D and 3D echocardiography. Circ Cardiovasc Imaging 2012;5(6):748–55.

39. Gruner C, Herzog B, Bettex D, et al. Quantification of mitral regurgitation by real time three-dimensional color Doppler flow echocardiography pre- and post-percutaneous mitral valve repair. Echocardiography 2015;32(7):1140–6.

40. Avenatti E, Mackensen GB, El-Tallawi KC, et al. Diagnostic value of 3-dimensional vena contracta area for the quantification of residual mitral regurgitation after MitraClip procedure. JACC Cardiovasc Interv 2019;12(6):582–91.

41. Ikenaga H, Hayashi A, Nagaura T, et al. Relation between pulmonary venous flow and left atrial pressure during percutaneous mitral valve repair with the MitraClip. Am J Cardiol 2018;122(8):1379–86.

42. Baumgartner H, Hung J, Bermejo J, et al. Echocardiographic assessment of valve stenosis: EAE/ASE recommendations for clinical practice. J Am Soc Echocardiogr 2009;22(1):1–23 [quiz: 101–2].

43. Estevez-Loureiro R, Franzen O, Winter R, et al. Echocardiographic and clinical outcomes of central versus noncentral percutaneous edge-to-edge repair of degenerative mitral regurgitation. J Am Coll Cardiol 2013;62(25):2370–7.

44. Mauri L, Garg P, Massaro JM, et al. The EVEREST II trial: design and rationale for a randomized study of the evalve mitraclip system compared with mitral valve surgery for mitral regurgitation. Am Heart J 2010;160(1):23–9.

45. Attizzani GF, Ohno Y, Capodanno D, et al. Extended use of percutaneous edge-to-edge mitral valve repair beyond EVEREST (Endovascular Valve Edge-to-Edge Repair) criteria: 30-day and 12-month clinical and echocardiographic outcomes from the GRASP (getting reduction of mitral insufficiency by percutaneous clip implantation) registry. JACC Cardiovasc Interv 2015;8(1 Pt A):74–82.

46. Taramasso M, Denti P, Latib A, et al. Clinical and anatomical predictors of MitraClip therapy failure for functional mitral regurgitation: single central clip strategy in asymmetric tethering. Int J Cardiol 2015;186:286–8.

47. Praz F, Braun D, Unterhuber M, et al. Edge-to-edge mitral valve repair with extended clip arms: early experience from a multicenter observational study. JACC Cardiovasc Interv 2019;12(14):1356–65.

Contemporary Management of Acute Decompensated Heart Failure and Cardiogenic Shock

Takeshi Kitai, MD, PhD[a,b,]*, Andrew Xanthopoulos, MD, PhD[c]

KEYWORDS

- Heart failure • Cardiogenic shock • Mechanical circulatory support

KEY POINTS

- Cardiogenic shock accounts for 5% of acute decompensated heart failure and is associated with high mortality and morbidity.
- Invasive monitoring using pulmonary artery catheter is useful in most cases of shock.
- Routine inotrope use is not supported by guidelines, but is essential in most patients with cardiogenic shock.
- Transcatheter intervention for severe aortic stenosis or severe mitral regurgitation may be beneficial in some patients.

INTRODUCTION

Cardiogenic shock (CS) is life-threatening condition characterized by end-organ hypoperfusion and hypoxia primarily due to cardiac dysfunction and a low cardiac output state.[1,2] CS is a complex and hemodynamically diverse state, and is conceptualized as a vicious cycle of cardiac injury, systemic deterioration, and further cardiac impairment. Despite the unacceptably high mortality and morbidity rates associated with CS, evidence or guidelines supporting optimal therapy for this entity are still limited.[3,4] Particularly, data regarding CS due to nonischemic etiologies are lacking because clinical trials have mainly focused on CS due to acute coronary syndrome (ACS), which is the most common etiology of CS.[1,5,6] Nonischemic etiologies of CS include severe

decompensation of chronic heart failure, valvular heart disease, myocarditis, or even Takotsubo syndrome.[7] Prompt diagnosis and early revascularization are key to the successful management of CS due to ACS, but nonischemic etiologies must also be rapidly diagnosed, and if present, managed appropriately.[8]

In patients with acute decompensated heart failure (ADHF), CS is the most severe form of presentation, accounting for less than 5% of ADHF.[7,9] However, the frequency of CS in ADHF varies depending on hospital type, with a higher frequency among hospitals that perform heart transplantation.[10] Despite significant advances in heart failure management and treatment, mortality among patients with ADHF presenting with CS remains substantially high.[3,4] Although the definition

[a] Department of Cardiovascular Medicine, Kobe City Medical Center General Hospital, 2-1-1 Minatojima-minamimachi, Chuo-ku, Kobe 650-0047, Japan; [b] Department of Clinical Research Support, Kobe City Medical Center General Hospital, 2-1-1 Minatojima-minamimachi, Chuo-ku, Kobe 650-0047, Japan; [c] Department of Cardiology, University General Hospital of Larissa, Larissa, Greece
* Corresponding author. Department of Cardiovascular Medicine, Kobe City Medical Center General Hospital, 2-1-1 Minatojima-minamimachi, Chuo-ku, Kobe 650-0047, Japan.
E-mail address: t-kitai@kcho.jp

Heart Failure Clin 16 (2020) 221–230
https://doi.org/10.1016/j.hfc.2019.12.005

of CS used in clinical trials and guidelines varies,[1,5,6] its contemporary definition in patients with ADHF is prolonged hypotension (systolic blood pressure <90 mm Hg or the need for vasopressors to increase blood pressure above 90 mm Hg) in the absence of hypovolemia or bleeding with signs of hypoperfusion. This review summarizes the challenges encountered in the diagnosis and management of CS in patients with ADHF.

HEMODYNAMIC MONITORING FOR CARDIOGENIC SHOCK

The treatment strategy for CS in ADHF should be carefully guided by hemodynamics assessment based on vital signs, physical examination, laboratory tests, echocardiography, and a more direct assessment via pulmonary artery catheterization (PAC), if needed. The most important point is that the goal of treatment for hypotensive patients with ADHF is to improve hypoperfusion, but not just to increase their blood pressure, because these patients with advanced heart failure (HF) may have a chronically low systolic blood pressure due to severe left ventricular (LV) systolic dysfunction. Therefore, it is crucial to promptly detect signs of hypoperfusion, such as cool extremities, tachycardia, and low urine output.

Laboratory biomarkers, such as serum lactate, are useful for assessing end-organ perfusion, and should be repeatedly monitored.[11] Elevated lactate levels are reflective of poor tissue perfusion, leading to increased production from anaerobic metabolism,[12,13] and they are associated with increased mortality in shock.[14] Although there is no clear cutoff value of lactate level for the definition of CS, serum lactate level greater than 2 or 4 mmol/L is generally considered to be elevated. Serum lactate can be serially measured to determine responses to therapies. In addition, echocardiography should be performed first immediately after presentation to evaluate the etiology of CS, and to assess cardiac function. Repetitive echocardiography should be used to monitor hemodynamic evolution. These monitoring procedures should be used even alongside invasive hemodynamic monitoring.

In this setting, invasive hemodynamic monitoring is a powerful tool for following a multidisciplinary approach involving procedural, mechanical, and pharmacologic interventions. Invasive hemodynamic monitoring using PAC should be considered in all patients with CS who do not respond to initial treatment or whose underlying hemodynamic status is uncertain[15,16]; however, its use should be limited to selected patients. The usefulness of PAC in critically ill patients is controversial because previous studies examining the utility of PAC for the measurement of cardiac output (CO) and pulmonary capillary wedge pressure failed to show any benefit regarding patient outcomes.[17,18] In addition to the information regarding intracardiac pressures and CO, several other parameters and indexes can be derived by the PAC use. Cardiac power output (CPO) is an index calculated as mean arterial pressure (MAP) × CO/451, and cardiac power index (CPI) is calculated as CPO divided by body surface area. These concepts indicate that the pumping ability of the heart can be quantified as the simultaneous product of flow (CO) and pressure (MAP). These parameters have been used as important measures of cardiac pumping function,[19] and are useful for diagnosis and as predictors of outcome in patients with ADHF and CS.[20–23] In the SHOCK Trial, CPO less than 0.53 and CPI less than 0.33 were identified as the strongest independent hemodynamic correlates of in-hospital mortality in CS.[24]

In summary, the assessment of hemodynamic status via the clinical examination, laboratory testing, echocardiographic examination, and PAC is mandatory in the management and better prognosis of patients with ADHF presenting with CS.

MANAGEMENT OF CARDIOGENIC SHOCK DUE TO HEART FAILURE
Pharmacotherapy

Inotropes such as dobutamine and milrinone can definitely improve hemodynamics in patients with ADHF and CS, if used appropriately. However, there is some concern that inotropic agents may adversely impact outcomes in patients with ADHF, with increasing heart rates and myocardial oxygen consumption leading to ischemia and/or arrhythmias. Several studies reported that inotropic agents are associated with worsening morbidity and mortality[25,26]; however, although positive evidence regarding inotropic therapy in CS is still limited, inotropic agents, including milrinone, dobutamine, and dopamine are commonly used for selected patients with CS to maintain systemic perfusion and preserve end-organ performance until definitive therapy is instituted or resolution of the acute precipitating problem occurs.[15]

Dobutamine
Dobutamine and milrinone are the most commonly used inotropes. Dobutamine acts primarily via β_1 receptors to increase cardiac contractility, producing peripheral vasodilation at lower concentrations and

vasocontraction at higher concentrations.[27] Although dobutamine has been shown to provide symptomatic relief in ADHF at low doses for a short duration,[28] long-term continuous infusion has been suggested to increase mortality,[29,30] in addition to the development of drug tolerance.[31] Combination therapy with dobutamine and milrinone causes a greater decrease in mean pulmonary artery pressure, pulmonary capillary wedge pressure, and systemic vascular resistance compared with dobutamine in patients with advanced HF.[32]

Milrinone

Milrinone is the most frequently used phosphodiesterase inhibitor. Phosphodiesterase inhibitors work downstream of adrenergic receptors within cardiomyocytes and vascular smooth muscle cells to inhibit the breakdown of cyclic adenosine monophosphate, leading to enhanced LV contractility and vasodilation. Milrinone produces less change in heart rate or cardiac oxygen consumption compared with dobutamine.[33,34] It decreases pulmonary artery pressures, broadening its potential indications in patients with coexisting pulmonary hypertension or right ventricular (RV) failure.[33,35] Given that milrinone bypasses β-adrenergic receptors to exert its affects, it may produce a stronger response in patients on β-blockers and induce less tolerance compared with the catecholaminergic inotropes.[34] Therefore, milrinone is theoretically a more favorable and effective drug than dobutamine in patients on chronic beta-blocker therapy. A retrospective study using the Acute Decompensated Heart Failure National Registry concluded that patients with dobutamine have higher in-hospital mortality compared with patients taking milrinone[36]; however, because of its vasodilator response, caution must be taken regarding its administration in patients with CS. Like dobutamine, the routine use of intravenous milrinone is currently not indicated in patients hospitalized with ADHF, because milrinone did not show a mortality benefit but was associated with increased rates of atrial arrhythmias and sustained hypotension requiring intervention.[37] In the OPTIME-CHF (Outcomes of a Prospective Trial of Intravenous Milrinone for Exacerbations of Chronic Heart Failure) trial, 949 hospitalized patients with ADHF were randomly assigned to a 48-hour to 72-hour infusion of milrinone or placebo. Milrinone therapy was associated with significant increase in hypotension requiring intervention and atrial arrhythmias, and with nonsignificant increase in mortality.[26] Thus, the routine use of inotropes in hospitalized patients with HF was found to be harmful,[25,26] and current guidelines recommend the judicious and short-term use of inotropic therapy only for carefully evaluated patients with ADHF complicated with CS.[16,27,28] Continuous monitoring of systemic and pulmonary vascular resistance with PAC may be a key to successful management of patients with hypotensive ADHF who receive milrinone. Milrinone also may be used in RV failure to augment RV performance via increased contractility. Milrinone decreases pulmonary vascular resistance more than dobutamine and is, thus, typically considered the inotrope of choice in RV failure due to high pulmonary afterload.[35]

Dopamine

Dopamine can provide inotropic and chronotropic effects when used at a moderate dosage (5–10 µg/kg per minute), whereas it can work predominantly as a vasopressor at higher dosages (>10–20 µg/kg per minute). The effect of dopamine in patients with ADHF was evaluated in the ROSE AHF (Renal Optimization Strategies Evaluation in Acute Heart Failure) trial, which noted no difference between low-dose dopamine, low-dose nesiritide, and placebo in diuresis or preservation of renal function in patients with ADHF and concomitant renal dysfunction.[36,38] The addition of low-dose dopamine to oral furosemide has similarly produced no difference in length of hospital stay, all-cause hospitalizations, or mortality, but the dopamine group had a more stable renal and electrolyte profile.[39] In a recent meta-analysis, low-dose dopamine improved renal function and diuresis but did not alter readmission rates or mortality.[40] However, because these trials excluded patients with CS, the use of dopamine in ADHF with CS should be individualized. Dopamine also may be used in RV failure to manage congestive hepatopathy or renal disease via splanchnic vasodilation.[41]

Vasopressors

Vasopressor therapy also can be used as a temporizing measure to preserve systemic blood pressure and end-organ perfusion.[16] Because there is the risk of increasing LV afterload and decreasing CO, vasopressor use should be limited in cases with persistent hypotension with symptoms or in the evidence of consequent end-organ hypoperfusion despite the optimization of filling pressures and seemingly appropriate use of inotropic agents. Vasopressors used in this setting include norepinephrine, high-dose dopamine (>5 µg/kg per minute), and vasopressin, and these should be carefully titrated to achieve adequate perfusion of vital organs. Dopamine and norepinephrine have β-inotropic as well as vasopressor activity.

Taken all together, although inotropes and vasopressors may improve hemodynamics in the short-term in patients with ADHF and CS, there is a concern that those agents may adversely impact outcomes in patients with ADHF leading to ischemia, arrhythmias, or even death.

Diuretics

Although many HF studies have not been able to demonstrate a mortality benefit with the use of diuretics, decongestion via diuretics remains a mainstay in the treatment of patients with ADHF who exhibit volume overload. However, the use of diuretics in patients with ADHF with CS remains challenging because it may further deteriorate hemodynamics and aggravate hypotension. Therefore, careful assessment of hemodynamics and optimal combination use of diuretics and vasoactive drugs are important in this scenario. PAC may serve as a tool for the accurate evaluation of hemodynamics. Ultrafiltration may be considered in patients with refractory diuretic resistance, as persistent volume overload after decongestive treatment is associated with worse outcomes.

Intervention for Critical Valve Disease

In patients presenting with ADHF and CS, prompt diagnosis and appropriate treatment of valvular dysfunction, such as calcified aortic stenosis and functional mitral regurgitation, is critical. Although morbidity and mortality remain high, recent advances in transcatheter structural heart intervention have the potential to improve outcomes in patients with shock and critical valvular lesions. However, careful patient selection, while balancing the benefits and risks, is needed.[42,43]

Aortic stenosis

Surgical aortic valve replacement (SAVR) remains the gold-standard treatment for symptomatic severe aortic stenosis (AS). Unfortunately, SAVR is not a good treatment option for patients with CS and severe AS due to extremely high operative risk.[44] We recently reported that acute decompensation due to severe AS was associated with an increased 5-year mortality compared with those with chronic HF or those without HF, even with SAVR.[45]

The introduction of transcatheter aortic valve replacement (TAVR) into clinical practice has revolutionized the management of AS. Although TAVR was initially offered as an alternative to SAVR in patients with a high risk for cardiac surgery, due to improvements in device technology, techniques, and success rates, TAVR has evolved into a relatively low-risk procedure despite the high comorbidity and relative frailty of target patients.[46–50] TAVR is also an attractive option for treating severe AS in patients with severe LV dysfunction, acute HF, and CS.[51] However, TAVR for high-risk patients with CS is still challenging. Recent reports revealed that TAVR in patients with CS due to decompensated AS was associated with a 30% mortality rate.[52,53] In addition to hemodynamic instability and systemic inflammatory response in patients with CS, difficulty in procedural planning because of limited information in an emergency case contributes to a worse prognosis. Multidetector computed tomography and transesophageal echocardiography are usually needed to measure annular dimensions and to determine the size of the TAVR prosthesis. In addition, the unavailability of important information like LV outflow tract calcification or annulus calcification may increase procedural risk. In a recent registry, urgent or emergency TAVR procedure was performed in 10% of cases, and severe LV dysfunction was observed in nearly 8% of cases.[54] Such patients may require mechanical circulatory support (MCS) devices before and/or during TAVR, such as intra-aortic balloon pumping (IABP), Impella, and veno-arterial extracorporeal membrane oxygenation (VA-ECMO) due to persistent hemodynamic deterioration.[55,56] Nonetheless, TAVR has the potential to markedly improve the hemodynamics leading to better survival. Further studies are needed to evaluate the safety and efficacy of TAVR in patients with CS and severe AS.

Mitral regurgitation

Severe functional mitral regurgitation is a common finding in patients with HF with systolic dysfunction. In patients with severe LV dysfunction and refractory CS, surgical mitral valve replacement or repair remains challenging because of its high operative mortality and morbidity.[57]

The MitraClip procedure is the most used interventional edge-to-edge repair transcatheter device and is a well-established treatment option for patients with severe mitral regurgitation who are at high risk for conventional surgical treatment.[58] However, currently, the MitraClip procedure is not recommended in patients with hemodynamic instability, including CS, or in those who need MCS.[59] Nevertheless, several recent case reports highlight the use of the MitraClip system as a rescue and/or salvage therapy in patients with refractory CS.[60–62] These reports have demonstrated that the MitraClip procedure can be performed safely in critically ill patients despite their potential need for inotropic or MCS support. Thus, MitraClip may assist in stabilizing critically ill patients and perhaps bridging them to more definitive surgical therapies or even transplantation. This indicates that the MitraClip procedure with or without MCS might be a rescue option for patients presenting with CS when stabilization by medical therapy before surgery is difficult or is not intended, although careful patient selection and mitral valve evaluation are essential.

Mechanical Circulatory Support

Because CS is characterized by an impaired CO followed by inadequate compensatory mechanisms and rapid deterioration leading to end-organ hypoperfusion and complete cardiovascular collapse,[2,63] MCS devices are an attractive therapeutic option in patients with CS because MCS can restore CO and normalize perfusion pressures (**Table 1**).[64] However, despite significant advancement with MCS devices, randomized trials have failed to show a mortality benefit with the use of these devices in CS.[1,65–68] As most of the patients enrolled in the trials mentioned earlier suffered from CS due to ACS, the effect of MCS for patients with ADHF and CS should be examined in future studies. MCS is also useful as a bridge to heart transplantation, which remains the gold-standard treatment for advanced HF, although heart transplantation is limited by the availability of transplant hearts for a growing population of patients with advanced and end-stage HF.

Intra-aortic balloon pumping

IABP has been one of the most widely used traditional MCS devices since the 1960s. IABP can increase coronary perfusion due to pump inflation at the onset of diastole, and decrease afterload, cardiac work, and myocardial oxygen consumption due to reduction in aortic end-diastolic and systolic pressures. However, although IABP was previously recommended as a class I indication in patients with CS, recent studies have questioned its potential benefit in CS. In the IABP-SHOCK II trial, 600 patients with acute myocardial infarction and CS were randomized to either IABP or medical therapy. IABP therapy failed to show any benefit regarding short-term or long-term survival.[1,69] As a result, the latest guidelines downgraded IABP use in patients with CS,[70–72] leading to decreasing IABP use.[73] There have been no data regarding IABP use for patients with ADHF with CS.

Extracorporeal membrane oxygenation

ECMO can provide biventricular support and respiratory support when combined with an oxygenator. Veno-venous ECMO is reserved for patients in isolated respiratory failure with no significant cardiac dysfunction, whereas VA-ECMO is considered in patients with cardiopulmonary collapse and is used to support patients in CS. Although adverse events are common and the rates of in-hospital mortality remain high in patients receiving ECMO,[74] VA-ECMO is a useful treatment option for patients with CS who are treated by an appropriate heart team in the presence of careful patient selection. The ELSO (Extracorporeal Life Support Organization) registry reported that ECMO use and the number of centers using ECMO are increasing.[74] However, the biggest hemodynamic limitation of VA-ECMO is its retrograde flow leading to increased LV afterload and inadequate LV decompression. Impella has been recently used to counteract this limitation of VA-ECMO.

Impella

Currently available percutaneous ventricular assist devices (VADs) include the nonpulsatile microaxial Impella 2.5, 5.0, and CP, and the Tandem Heart. Compared with IABP, percutaneous LV assist devices were associated with a higher cardiac index, higher MAP, and lower pulmonary capillary wedge pressure but increased bleeding complications. No difference was observed in 30-day mortality.[75] In the USpella Registry, the use of Impella 2.5 before percutaneous coronary intervention showed more complete revascularizations and improved survival compared with IABP in the setting of refractory CS complicating ACS.[76] However, in another randomized trial enrolling patients with CS complicating ACS, Impella CP was not associated with decreased 30-day mortality compared with IABP.[77] The combination therapy with VA-ECMO and Impella, named ECPella, which can offer LV unloading and reduce LV afterload and, hence, pulmonary edema,[78] should be evaluated in future studies.

CentriMag

CentriMag is a surgically implanted temporary MCS device, and was the first implantable VAD with biventricular capability approved by the Food and Drug Administration.[79] This system is typically implanted via median sternotomy. Recently, Takeda and colleagues[80] developed a minimally invasive surgical approach combining ECMO with CentriMag VAD for short-term CS treatment. The major advantage of this system in addition to full hemodynamic support is the ability to add an oxygenator to the right side of the configuration, thus, providing complete right, left, and pulmonary support. This system showed noninferior 30-day and overall 1-year survival versus CentriMag BiVAD alone, but eliminated the need for cardiopulmonary bypass and reduced blood product utilization, as well as the bleeding events.

Table 1
Characteristics and hemodynamic effects of temporary mechanical circulatory support devices

MCS devices	IABP	Impella 2.5	Impella CP	Impella 5.0	Peripheral VA-ECMO
Pump mechanism	Pneumatic	Axial flow	Axial flow	Axial flow	Centrifugal
Cannula, Fr	8	13	14	23	13.5–17 (outflow)
Hemodynamic support, L/min	0–1	2.5	3–4	5	3–6
Insertion	Percutaneous: descending aorta via femoral artery	Percutaneous: femoral artery retrograde across aortic valve	Percutaneous: femoral artery retrograde across aortic valve	Surgical cutdown: subclavian artery retrograde across aortic valve	Percutaneous or surgical: femoral vein (inflow) and femoral artery (outflow)
LV preload	Slightly reduced	Slightly reduced	Slightly reduced	Slightly reduced	Reduced
LV afterload	Reduced	Neutral	Neutral	Neutral	Increased
PCWP	Slightly reduced	Reduced	Reduced	Reduced	Variable
LV stroke volume	Slight increase	Neutral	Neutral	Neutral	Reduced
Peripheral tissue perfusion	No significant increase	Improved	Improved	Improved	Improved
Hemolysis	+	+++	++	+	++
Bleeding	–	+	+	++	+++
Limb ischemia	+	++	++	++	++
Cost	+	+++	+++	+++	++

Abbreviations: IABP, intra-aortic balloon pumping; LV, left ventricular; MCS, mechanical circulatory support; PCWP, pulmonary capillary wedge pressure; VA-ECMO, veno-arterial extracorporeal membrane oxygenation.

Hemodynamic support for right ventricle

Isolated RV failure has become more recognized in recent times, leading to the development of devices specific for this cardiac dysfunction. RV dysfunction may occur in isolation or in combination with LV dysfunction. That MCS devices can improve hemodynamics without impacting mortality is because MCS therapy mainly focuses only on supporting the LV, while leaving the RV unaddressed. The Impella RP is designed for univentricular RV support. The Impella RP is an intracardiac microaxial blood pump designed for the management of RV failure and can be inserted through the femoral vein. The prospective RECOVER RIGHT study showed that this safe, easily deployed, and reliable pump resulted in immediate hemodynamic benefit in patients with life-threatening RV failure, leading to its approval for use through a humanitarian device exemption.[81]

Few clinical studies have evaluated inotropes in the setting of primary RV failure. At low doses, dobutamine improves RV–pulmonary artery coupling via reduced pulmonary vascular resistance and increased RV contractility.[82]

SUMMARY

The severe decompensation of chronic HF may lead to CS. The diagnostic approach of these patients includes the assessment of vital signs, physical examination, laboratory tests, echocardiography, and sometimes hemodynamic evaluation by PAC. Despite the controversy surrounding their benefits, the use of inotropes, vasopressors, and MCS is needed in carefully selected patients presenting with ADHF and CS. Along with technological advances, superior percutaneous MCS devices, a promising therapeutic option, are predicted to become more commercially available in the future.

DISCLOSURE

The authors have nothing to disclose.

REFERENCES

1. Thiele H, Zeymer U, Neumann FJ, et al. Intraaortic balloon support for myocardial infarction with cardiogenic shock. N Engl J Med 2012;367: 1287–96.

2. Reynolds HR, Hochman JS. Cardiogenic shock: current concepts and improving outcomes. Circulation 2008;117:686–97.

3. Stretch R, Sauer CM, Yuh DD, et al. National trends in the utilization of short-term mechanical circulatory support: incidence, outcomes, and cost analysis. J Am Coll Cardiol 2014;64:1407–15.

4. Goldberg RJ, Makam RC, Yarzebski J, et al. Decade-long trends (2001-2011) in the incidence and hospital death rates associated with the in-hospital development of cardiogenic shock after acute myocardial infarction. Circ Cardiovasc Qual Outcomes 2016;9:117–25.

5. Hochman JS, Sleeper LA, Webb JG, et al. Early revascularization in acute myocardial infarction complicated by cardiogenic shock. SHOCK investigators. should we emergently revascularize occluded coronaries for cardiogenic shock. N Engl J Med 1999;341:625–34.

6. Ponikowski P, Voors AA, Anker SD, et al. 2016 ESC guidelines for the diagnosis and treatment of acute and chronic heart failure: the task force for the diagnosis and treatment of acute and chronic heart failure of the European Society of Cardiology (ESC). Developed with the special contribution of the Heart Failure Association (HFA) of the ESC. Eur Heart J 2016;37:2129–200.

7. Harjola VP, Lassus J, Sionis A, et al. Clinical picture and risk prediction of short-term mortality in cardiogenic shock. Eur J Heart Fail 2015;17:501–9.

8. Hochman JS, Buller CE, Sleeper LA, et al. Cardiogenic shock complicating acute myocardial infarction–etiologies, management and outcome: a report from the SHOCK trial registry. SHould we emergently revascularize Occluded Coronaries for cardiogenic shocK? J Am Coll Cardiol 2000;36: 1063–70.

9. Nieminen MS, Brutsaert D, Dickstein K, et al. EuroHeart Failure Survey II (EHFS II): a survey on hospitalized acute heart failure patients: description of population. Eur Heart J 2006;27:2725–36.

10. Adams KF Jr, Fonarow GC, Emerman CL, et al. Characteristics and outcomes of patients hospitalized for heart failure in the United States: rationale, design, and preliminary observations from the first 100,000 cases in the acute decompensated heart failure national registry (ADHERE). Am Heart J 2005;149:209–16.

11. Cecconi M, De Backer D, Antonelli M, et al. Consensus on circulatory shock and hemodynamic monitoring. Task force of the European Society of Intensive Care Medicine. Intensive Care Med 2014; 40:1795–815.

12. Kraut JA, Madias NE. Lactic acidosis. N Engl J Med 2014;371:2309–19.

13. Levraut J, Ciebiera JP, Chave S, et al. Mild hyperlactatemia in stable septic patients is due to impaired lactate clearance rather than overproduction. Am J Respir Crit Care Med 1998;157:1021–6.

14. del Portal DA, Shofer F, Mikkelsen ME, et al. Emergency department lactate is associated with mortality in older adults admitted with and without infections. Acad Emerg Med 2010;17:260–8.

15. Writing Committee Members, Yancy CW, Jessup M, Bozkurt B, et al. 2013 ACCF/AHA guideline for the management of heart failure: a report of the American College of Cardiology Foundation/American Heart Association task force on practice guidelines. Circulation 2013;128: e240–327.

16. McMurray JJ, Adamopoulos S, Anker SD, et al. ESC guidelines for the diagnosis and treatment of acute and chronic heart failure 2012: the task force for the diagnosis and treatment of acute and chronic heart failure 2012 of the European Society of Cardiology. Developed in collaboration with the Heart Failure Association (HFA) of the ESC. Eur Heart J 2012; 33:1787–847.

17. Connors AF Jr, Speroff T, Dawson NV, et al. The effectiveness of right heart catheterization in the initial care of critically ill patients. SUPPORT investigators. JAMA 1996;276:889–97.

18. Zion MM, Balkin J, Rosenmann D, et al. Use of pulmonary artery catheters in patients with acute myocardial infarction. Analysis of experience in 5,841 patients in the SPRINT registry. SPRINT study group. Chest 1990;98:1331–5.

19. Cotter G, Williams SG, Vered Z, et al. Role of cardiac power in heart failure. Curr Opin Cardiol 2003;18: 215–22.

20. Cotter G, Moshkovitz Y, Kaluski E, et al. The role of cardiac power and systemic vascular resistance in the pathophysiology and diagnosis of patients with acute congestive heart failure. Eur J Heart Fail 2003;5:443–51.

21. Tan LB, Littler WA. Measurement of cardiac reserve in cardiogenic shock: implications for prognosis and management. Br Heart J 1990;64:121–8.

22. Cohen-Solal A, Tabet JY, Logeart D, et al. A non-invasively determined surrogate of cardiac power ('circulatory power') at peak exercise is a powerful

prognostic factor in chronic heart failure. Eur Heart J 2002;23:806–14.

23. Williams SG, Cooke GA, Wright DJ, et al. Peak exercise cardiac power output; a direct indicator of cardiac function strongly predictive of prognosis in chronic heart failure. Eur Heart J 2001;22: 1496–503.

24. Fincke R, Hochman JS, Lowe AM, et al. Cardiac power is the strongest hemodynamic correlate of mortality in cardiogenic shock: a report from the SHOCK trial registry. J Am Coll Cardiol 2004;44:340–8.

25. Felker GM, Benza RL, Chandler AB, et al. Heart failure etiology and response to milrinone in decompensated heart failure: results from the OPTIME-CHF study. J Am Coll Cardiol 2003;41:997–1003.

26. Cuffe MS, Califf RM, Adams KF Jr, et al. Short-term intravenous milrinone for acute exacerbation of chronic heart failure: a randomized controlled trial. JAMA 2002;287:1541–7.

27. Hunt SA, Abraham WT, Chin MH, et al. 2009 focused update incorporated into the ACC/AHA 2005 guidelines for the diagnosis and management of heart failure in adults: a report of the American College of Cardiology Foundation/American Heart Association task force on practice guidelines developed in collaboration with the International Society for Heart and Lung Transplantation. J Am Coll Cardiol 2009; 53:e1–90.

28. Heart Failure Society of America, Lindenfeld J, Albert NM, Boehmer JP, et al. HFSA 2010 comprehensive heart failure practice guideline. J Card Fail 2010;16:e1–194.

29. Tuttle RR, Mills J. Dobutamine: development of a new catecholamine to selectively increase cardiac contractility. Circ Res 1975;36:185–96.

30. Patel MB, Kaplan IV, Patni RN, et al. Sustained improvement in flow-mediated vasodilation after short-term administration of dobutamine in patients with severe congestive heart failure. Circulation 1999;99:60–4.

31. Stevenson LW. Inotropic therapy for heart failure. N Engl J Med 1998;339:1848–50.

32. O'Connor CM, Gattis WA, Uretsky BF, et al. Continuous intravenous dobutamine is associated with an increased risk of death in patients with advanced heart failure: insights from the Flolan International Randomized Survival Trial (FIRST). Am Heart J 1999;138:78–86.

33. Unverferth DA, Blanford M, Kates RE, et al. Tolerance to dobutamine after a 72 hour continuous infusion. Am J Med 1980;69:262–6.

34. Yamani MH, Haji SA, Starling RC, et al. Comparison of dobutamine-based and milrinone-based therapy for advanced decompensated congestive heart failure: hemodynamic efficacy, clinical outcome, and economic impact. Am Heart J 2001;142:998–1002.

35. Grose R, Strain J, Greenberg M, et al. Systemic and coronary effects of intravenous milrinone and dobutamine in congestive heart failure. J Am Coll Cardiol 1986;7:1107–13.

36. Abraham WT, Adams KF, Fonarow GC, et al. In-hospital mortality in patients with acute decompensated heart failure requiring intravenous vasoactive medications: an analysis from the acute decompensated heart failure national registry (ADHERE). J Am Coll Cardiol 2005;46:57–64.

37. Eichhorn EJ, Konstam MA, Weiland DS, et al. Differential effects of milrinone and dobutamine on right ventricular preload, afterload and systolic performance in congestive heart failure secondary to ischemic or idiopathic dilated cardiomyopathy. Am J Cardiol 1987;60:1329–33.

38. King JB, Shah RU, Sainski-Nguyen A, et al. Effect of inpatient dobutamine versus milrinone on out-of-hospital mortality in patients with acute decompensated heart failure. Pharmacotherapy 2017;37: 662–72.

39. Chen HH, Anstrom KJ, Givertz MM, et al. Low-dose dopamine or low-dose nesiritide in acute heart failure with renal dysfunction: the ROSE acute heart failure randomized trial. JAMA 2013; 310:2533–43.

40. Wan SH, Stevens SR, Borlaug BA, et al. Differential response to low-dose dopamine or low-dose nesiritide in acute heart failure with reduced or preserved ejection fraction: results from the ROSE AHF trial (Renal Optimization Strategies Evaluation in Acute Heart Failure). Circ Heart Fail 2016;9(8) [pii: e002593].

41. Giamouzis G, Butler J, Starling RC, et al. Impact of dopamine infusion on renal function in hospitalized heart failure patients: results of the Dopamine in Acute Decompensated Heart Failure (DAD-HF) Trial. J Card Fail 2010;16:922–30.

42. Xing F, Hu X, Jiang J, et al. A meta-analysis of low-dose dopamine in heart failure. Int J Cardiol 2016; 222:1003–11.

43. Asgar AW, Mack MJ, Stone GW. Secondary mitral regurgitation in heart failure: pathophysiology, prognosis, and therapeutic considerations. J Am Coll Cardiol 2015;65:1231–48.

44. Luscher TF. Frontiers of valvular heart disease: from aortic stenosis to the tricuspid valve and congenital anomalies. Eur Heart J 2017;38:611–4.

45. Carabello BA, Green LH, Grossman W, et al. Hemodynamic determinants of prognosis of aortic valve replacement in critical aortic stenosis and advanced congestive heart failure. Circulation 1980;62:42–8.

46. Nagao K, Taniguchi T, Morimoto T, et al. Acute heart failure in patients with severe aortic stenosis—insights from the CURRENT AS registry. Circ J 2018; 82:874–85.

47. Leon MB, Smith CR, Mack M, et al. Transcatheter aortic-valve implantation for aortic stenosis in patients who cannot undergo surgery. N Engl J Med 2010;363:1597–607.

48. Leon MB, Smith CR, Mack MJ, et al. Transcatheter or surgical aortic-valve replacement in intermediate-risk patients. N Engl J Med 2016;374:1609–20.

49. Thourani VH, Kodali S, Makkar RR, et al. Transcatheter aortic valve replacement versus surgical valve replacement in intermediate-risk patients: a propensity score analysis. Lancet 2016;387:2218–25.

50. Afilalo J, Lauck S, Kim DH, et al. Frailty in older adults undergoing aortic valve replacement: the FRAILTY-AVR study. J Am Coll Cardiol 2017;70:689–700.

51. Mack MJ, Leon MB, Thourani VH, et al. Transcatheter aortic-valve replacement with a balloon-expandable valve in low-risk patients. N Engl J Med 2019;380:1695–705.

52. Holmes DR Jr, Mack MJ, Kaul S, et al. 2012 ACCF/AATS/SCAI/STS expert consensus document on transcatheter aortic valve replacement: developed in collaboration with the American Heart Association, American Society of Echocardiography, European Association for Cardio-Thoracic Surgery, Heart Failure Society of America, Mended Hearts, Society of Cardiovascular Anesthesiologists, Society of Cardiovascular Computed Tomography, and Society for Cardiovascular Magnetic Resonance. Catheter Cardiovasc Interv 2012;79:1023–82.

53. Frerker C, Schewel J, Schluter M, et al. Emergency transcatheter aortic valve replacement in patients with cardiogenic shock due to acutely decompensated aortic stenosis. EuroIntervention 2016;11:1530–6.

54. Landes U, Orvin K, Codner P, et al. Urgent transcatheter aortic valve implantation in patients with severe aortic stenosis and acute heart failure: procedural and 30-day outcomes. Can J Cardiol 2016;32:726–31.

55. Holmes DR Jr, Nishimura RA, Grover FL, et al. Annual outcomes with transcatheter valve therapy: from the STS/ACC TVT registry. Ann Thorac Surg 2016;101:789–800.

56. Singh V, Damluji AA, Mendirichaga R, et al. Elective or emergency use of mechanical circulatory support devices during transcatheter aortic valve replacement. J Interv Cardiol 2016;29:513–22.

57. Singh V, Patel SV, Savani C, et al. Mechanical circulatory support devices and transcatheter aortic valve implantation (from the national inpatient sample). Am J Cardiol 2015;116:1574–80.

58. Fasol R, Lakew F, Wetter S. Mitral repair in patients with a ruptured papillary muscle. Am Heart J 2000;139:549–54.

59. Feldman T, Foster E, Glower DD, et al. Percutaneous repair or surgery for mitral regurgitation. N Engl J Med 2011;364:1395–406.

60. Tamburino C, Ussia GP, Maisano F, et al. Percutaneous mitral valve repair with the MitraClip system: acute results from a real world setting. Eur Heart J 2010;31:1382–9.

61. Tarsia G, Smaldone C, Costantino MF. Effective percutaneous "edge-to-edge" mitral valve repair with mitraclip in a patient with acute post-MI regurgitation not related to papillary muscle rupture. Catheter Cardiovasc Interv 2016;88:1177–80.

62. Bilge M, Alemdar R, Yasar AS. Successful percutaneous mitral valve repair with the MitraClip system of acute mitral regurgitation due to papillary muscle rupture as complication of acute myocardial infarction. Catheter Cardiovasc Interv 2014;83:E137–40.

63. Pleger ST, Chorianopoulos E, Krumsdorf U, et al. Percutaneous edge-to-edge repair of mitral regurgitation as a bail-out strategy in critically ill patients. J Invasive Cardiol 2013;25:69–72.

64. Califf RM, Bengtson JR. Cardiogenic shock. N Engl J Med 1994;330:1724–30.

65. Burkhoff D. Device therapy: where next in cardiogenic shock owing to myocardial infarction? Nat Rev Cardiol 2015;12:383–4.

66. Thiele H, Sick P, Boudriot E, et al. Randomized comparison of intra-aortic balloon support with a percutaneous left ventricular assist device in patients with revascularized acute myocardial infarction complicated by cardiogenic shock. Eur Heart J 2005;26:1276–83.

67. Burkhoff D, Cohen H, Brunckhorst C, et al, Tandem-Heart Investigators Group. A randomized multicenter clinical study to evaluate the safety and efficacy of the TandemHeart percutaneous ventricular assist device versus conventional therapy with intraaortic balloon pumping for treatment of cardiogenic shock. Am Heart J 2006;152:469.e1-8.

68. Seyfarth M, Sibbing D, Bauer I, et al. A randomized clinical trial to evaluate the safety and efficacy of a percutaneous left ventricular assist device versus intra-aortic balloon pumping for treatment of cardiogenic shock caused by myocardial infarction. J Am Coll Cardiol 2008;52:1584–8.

69. Ouweneel DM, Eriksen E, Sjauw KD, et al. Percutaneous mechanical circulatory support versus intra-aortic balloon pump in cardiogenic shock after acute myocardial infarction. J Am Coll Cardiol 2017;69:278–87.

70. Thiele H, Zeymer U, Neumann FJ, et al. Intra-aortic balloon counterpulsation in acute myocardial infarction complicated by cardiogenic shock (IABP-SHOCK II): final 12 month results of a randomised, open-label trial. Lancet 2013;382:1638–45.

71. Kolh P, Windecker S, Alfonso F, et al. 2014 ESC/EACTS guidelines on myocardial revascularization: the task force on Myocardial Revascularization of the European Society of Cardiology (ESC) and the European Association for Cardio-Thoracic Surgery

(EACTS). Developed with the special contribution of the European Association of Percutaneous Cardiovascular Interventions (EAPCI). Eur J Cardiothorac Surg 2014;46:517–92.

72. O'Gara PT, Kushner FG, Ascheim DD, et al. 2013 ACCF/AHA guideline for the management of ST-elevation myocardial infarction: executive summary: a report of the American College of Cardiology Foundation/American Heart Association task force on practice guidelines. Circulation 2013;127: 529–55.

73. Ibanez B, James S, Agewall S, et al. 2017 ESC guidelines for the management of acute myocardial infarction in patients presenting with ST-segment elevation: the task force for the management of acute myocardial infarction in patients presenting with ST-segment elevation of the European Society of Cardiology (ESC). Eur Heart J 2018;39:119–77.

74. Kilic A, Shukrallah BN, Kilic A, et al. Initiation and management of adult veno-arterial extracorporeal life support. Ann Transl Med 2017;5:67.

75. Thiagarajan RR, Barbaro RP, Rycus PT, et al. Extracorporeal life support organization registry international report 2016. ASAIO J 2017;63:60–7.

76. O'Neill WW, Schreiber T, Wohns DH, et al. The current use of Impella 2.5 in acute myocardial infarction complicated by cardiogenic shock: results from the USpella registry. J Interv Cardiol 2014; 27:1–11.

77. Ouweneel DM, Eriksen E, Seyfarth M, et al. Percutaneous mechanical circulatory support versus intra-aortic balloon pump for treating cardiogenic shock: meta-analysis. J Am Coll Cardiol 2017;69: 358–60.

78. Koeckert MS, Jorde UP, Naka Y, et al. Impella LP 2.5 for left ventricular unloading during venoarterial extracorporeal membrane oxygenation support. J Card Surg 2011;26:666–8.

79. Slaughter MS, Rogers JG, Milano CA, et al. Advanced heart failure treated with continuous-flow left ventricular assist device. N Engl J Med 2009; 361:2241–51.

80. Takeda K, Garan AR, Ando M, et al. Minimally invasive CentriMag ventricular assist device support integrated with extracorporeal membrane oxygenation in cardiogenic shock patients: a comparison with conventional CentriMag biventricular support configuration. Eur J Cardiothorac Surg 2017;52:1055–61.

81. Anderson MB, Goldstein J, Milano C, et al. Benefits of a novel percutaneous ventricular assist device for right heart failure: the prospective RECOVER RIGHT study of the Impella RP device. J Heart Lung Transplant 2015;34:1549–60.

82. Kerbaul F, Rondelet B, Motte S, et al. Effects of norepinephrine and dobutamine on pressure load-induced right ventricular failure. Crit Care Med 2004;32:1035–40.

Acute and Chronic Effects of Cancer Drugs on the Cardiovascular System

Shohei Moriyama, MD*, Mitsuhiro Fukata, MD, Hitoshi Kusaba, MD,
Toru Maruyama, MD, Koichi Akashi, MD

KEYWORDS

- Cardiotoxicity • Cardio-oncology • CTRCD • Trastuzumab • Anthracycline
- Hematopoietic stem cell transplantation • GVHD

KEY POINTS

- Cancer and cardiovascular disease (CVD) share risk factors and many patients with cancer have clinical or subclinical CVD at the time of cancer diagnosis.
- During and after cardiotoxic therapy, periodic cardiac examinations are important to detect any cancer therapy–related cardiac dysfunction (CTRCD).
- CTRCD can be ameliorated; however, discontinuation of heart failure drugs could lead to worsening of heart failure in CTRCD patients.
- Hematopoietic stem cell transplantation can provoke cardiotoxicity because of cancer drug toxicity and graft-versus-host disease (GVHD).

INTRODUCTION

Long-term survival rate in patients with cancer has been increased by the development of novel anti-cancer agents and radiation therapy. However, morbidity and mortality because of adverse effects of cancer therapy have also increased. In particular, cardiovascular damage is a frequent side effect that can potentially lead to fatal events in patients with cancer, and the development of new treatments can result in unknown cardiotoxicity.[1–3] In addition, the proportion of older patients with cancer and survivors has increased exponentially, and cardiovascular diseases (CVD) are prevalent in these elderly patients with cancer.[4] Cancer and CVD share risk factors (ie, smoking, obesity, diabetes, and hypertension); therefore, many patients with cancer have clinical or subclinical CVD at the time of cancer diagnosis. Cancer therapy has to be modified in patients with cancer with

CVD to avoid severe cardiotoxicity. This is because cardiotoxicity observed during cancer therapy may result in interruption of cancer treatment or use of a suboptimal regimen. Even if clinically overt CVD is not evident, CVD risk factors frequently worsen during cancer therapy and increase the incidence of future CVD, leading to poor oncologic outcomes.[5,6] In fact, the cumulative primary cause of death over 10 years' follow-up in breast cancer survivors was CVD.[7] CVD and its associated risk factors also increase for patients without risk factors at the time of cancer diagnosis. The cumulative incidence of life-threatening chronic disorders exceeds 40% in childhood cancer survivors at 30 years after cancer diagnosis.[8,9] From this point of view, consideration of comorbidity, especially CVD, is important not only during, but also after the period of cancer therapy, and CVD risk management can help to

Sources of Funding: This work was supported by JSPS KAKENHI Grant Number JP17K11577.
Department of Hematology, Oncology and Cardiovascular Medicine, Kyushu University Hospital, Maidashi 3-1-1, Higashi-ku, Fukuoka 812-8582, Japan
* Corresponding author.
E-mail address: s-mori@med.kyushu-u.ac.jp

improve the overall survival of patients with cancer. This report describes the acute and chronic effects of cancer therapy on the cardiovascular system by presenting representative cases showing heart failure caused by anticancer drugs and therapy.

CASE 1

A 58-year-old woman with breast cancer (cT1N1M0 stage IIA, estrogen receptor-positive, progesterone receptor-negative, and HER2-positive) was treated with paclitaxel, 80 mg/m^2, and trastuzumab, 4 mg/kg, as a neoadjuvant chemotherapy. She had hypertension but no other common risk factors for CVD, and had no family histories of CVD. Pretreatment cardiac function was within the normal range, and no valvular diseases were detected. Left ventricular ejection fraction (LVEF) was 63.4%, and LV end-diastolic diameter (LVDd) and end-systolic diameter (LVDs) were 48 mm and 31 mm, respectively. Four months after the initiation of chemotherapy, she complained of orthopnea and exertional dyspnea, which was consistent with New York Heart Association functional class III congestive heart failure. Transthoracic echocardiogram (TTE) revealed severe mitral regurgitation (MR) and severe tricuspid regurgitation associated with diffuse LV dysfunction, that is, LVEF, LVDd, and LVDs were 34.4%, 54 mm, and 45 mm, respectively. No coronary artery stenosis was detected by angiography, and cardiac MRI indicated diffuse LV dysfunction and myocardial interstitial fibrosis. The patient was clinically diagnosed as trastuzumab-related cardiomyopathy. Chemotherapy was suspended and treatment of heart failure with diuretic, inotropic, and vasodilatory agents was started. Administration of enalapril, which was switched to candesartan because of intolerance, bisoprolol, and spironolactone was initiated. After recovery of the decompensated heart failure, an aromatase inhibitors and subsequent estrogen antagonist as the second-line of breast cancer treatment were also administered because she did not want a mastectomy.

Twenty-one months after cessation of trastuzumab, her cardiac function completely recovered to a baseline level of LVEF of 66.1% associated with a low brain natriuretic peptide of 5.8 pg/mL. TTE presented reverse cardiac remodeling (LVDd and LVDs 46 mm and 29 mm, respectively). In addition, MR and tricuspid regurgitation were also reduced to a low level, and administration of spironolactone was discontinued. However, 9 months after the discontinuation of spironolactone, heart failure was re-exacerbated at New York Heart Association functional class III with an LVEF of 20.1% and brain natriuretic peptide of 1754 pg/mL. Catheter examination revealed intact coronary arteries and Forrester class IV hemodynamics (mean pulmonary capillary wedge pressure, 35 mm Hg; cardiac index, 2.06 mL/min/m^2). The intensification of medications for heart failure including reinitiation of spironolactone, titration of bisoprolol and candesartan, and administration of digoxin improved LV function (**Table 1**). Although the LV functional recovery was not complete (LVEF at 4 months after re-exacerbation was at most 44.3%), because of heart failure control, it was possible to reinitiate trastuzumab chemotherapy without heart failure exacerbation when the breast cancer progressed.

CASE 2

A 64-year-old man with a long-standing history of atrial fibrillation (AF) and chronic heart failure from the age of 50 years was diagnosed with esophageal stenosis after endoscopic submucosal dissection for esophageal cancer. The patient was followed up by computed tomography scanning that incidentally detected a right atrial tumor. Urgent right atrial tumor resection, tricuspid valve annuloplasty, and left atrial appendage closure were performed to avoid a pulmonary tumor embolism. A Ewing sarcoma was identified pathologically by the detection of EWSR1 gene mutation and overexpression of CD99, vimentin, and CD56. Alternating vincristine, doxorubicin, cyclophosphamide, and ifosfamide, etoposide (VDC/IE)-based multimodality therapy was selected based on the standard treatment of Ewing sarcoma. Pretreatment LV systolic function was within the normal range; the LVEF was 64.0% and LVDd, LVDs, intraventricular septum thickness, and posterior wall thickness were 48.2 mm, 31.6 mm, 10 mm, and 10 mm, respectively. Long-standing AF had caused left atrial dilatation (left atrial volume index, 91.6 mL/m^2) and mild to moderate MR without pulmonary hypertension. Bisoprolol was prescribed for AF rate control, but other heart failure treatment options, such as an angiotensin-converting enzyme inhibitor, were not administered because he had normal LV systolic function. No clinical complications other than myelosuppression and febrile neutropenia were observed until the fourth course of VDC/IE. Before starting the fifth course of chemotherapy, TTE revealed a slightly impaired LV systolic function with LVEF 56.8%; however, troponin-T was lower than the detection range and there was no symptomatic heart failure, so the fifth course was started. However, troponin-T was slightly elevated

Table 1
Case 1: acute and re-exacerbated heart failure related to trastuzumab

	Pretreatment	At the Time of Decompensated Heart Failure	6 mo After Trastuzumab Cessation	20 mo After Trastuzumab Cessation	Heart Failure Re-exacerbation (9 mo After Spironolactone Cessation)	4 mo After Heart Failure Re-exacerbation
Echocardiogram						
LVEF (%)	63	34	41	66	20	44
LVDd (mm)	48	54	42	46	56	47
LVDs (mm)	31	45	33	29	51	37
IVS (mm)	8	8	9	8	8	9
PW (mm)	8	8	9	8	10	9
E/A	0.85	1.50	0.50	0.80	0.5	0.7
DcT (ms)	160	85	238	259	158	250
E/E'	6.4	10.3	10.8	9.0	13.2	11.7
Laboratory data						
BNP		233.0	12.5	5.8	1754.7	8.3
Medication						
Breast cancer	Paclitaxel and trastuzumab	Cessation of paclitaxel and trastuzumab Initiation of hormonal therapy				
HF		Initiation of enalapril (exchanged to candesartan), bisoprolol, and spironolactone		Discontinuation of spironolactone	Reinitiation of spironolactone Titration of bisoprolol and candesartan Administration of digoxin	Reinitiation of trastuzumab

Abbreviations: BNP, brain natriuretic peptide; DcT, deceleration time; HF, heart failure; IVS, interventricular septum; PW, posterior left ventricular wall.

on Day 3 (0.015 ng/mL) and LV function was exacerbated, that is, LVEF, LVDd, and LVDs were 44.4%, 54 mm, and 42 mm on TTE after completion of the fifth course of VDC therapy. There was no evidence of late gadolinium enhancement on cardiac MRI, and LVEF was ameliorated at 52.8% before the sixth course of chemotherapy because of the administration of enalapril and eplerenone (serial changes of the TTE parameters are described in **Table 2**). Subsequent chemotherapy that did not include doxorubicin could be administered safely under concurrent heart failure treatment. At follow-up, he was living an ordinary life without symptomatic heart failure or recurrence of cardiac sarcoma.

CASE 3

A 52-year-old woman was diagnosed with follicular lymphoma and was treated with eight courses of R-CHOP, a combined therapy of rituximab, cyclophosphamide, doxorubicin, vincristine, and prednisone. After the first-line chemotherapy, the disease relapsed and six courses of combination chemotherapy with bendamustine and rituximab was administered. However, the disease relapsed a second time and she received an allogenic peripheral blood stem cell transplantation. Pretransplant TTE showed normal cardiac function and no valvular disease, that is, LVEF was 64.8%.

LVDd and LVDs were 40 mm and 24 mm, respectively, despite high-dose doxorubicin of 400 mg/m. The donor was her son and her HLA matched her son's HLA 7/8, indicating one local mismatch of HLA-DR. The conditioning regimen was fludarabine, melphalan, and 2 Gy total body irradiation, and graft versus-host disease (GVHD) prophylaxis was performed using tacrolimus and short-term methotrexate. Febrile neutropenia developed early after transplantation, but ameliorated with antibiotics, and neutrophil engraftment occurred at Day 21 after transplantation without acute GVHD of the skin, gut, or liver. However, body weight gradually increased and pleural effusion appeared. Fluid retention was refractory to diuretics, and kidney function also showed exacerbation. The patient complained of fatigue and her jugular vein was distended. TTE revealed pericardial effusion (PE) with right atrial and ventricular collapse and mildly impaired LV systolic function (LVEF of 55%). Pericardial puncture was performed at Day 49 for diagnosis and treatment of heart failure. Immediately after pericardiocentesis, her body weight decreased and renal function was ameliorated (serial change of the TTE parameter is described in **Table 3**). No bacteria count and class 2 cytology led us to a diagnosis of pericardial GVHD, and prednisone was initiated. Re-exacerbation of PE was not confirmed, and she was discharged on Day 91.

Table 2
Case 2: CTRCD caused by anthracycline and partial amelioration after heart failure therapy

	Pretreatment	Before Fifth Course of VDC/ IE Therapy (Total DXR 270 mg/m^2)	After Completion of Fifth Course VDC Therapy (Total DXR 330 mg/m^2)	Before Sixth Course of VDC/ IE Therapy (Total DXR 330 mg/m^2)	6 mo After Completion of Total VDC/IE Therapy (Total DXR 330 mg/m^2)
Echocardiogram					
LVEF (%)	64	57	44	53	53
LVDd (mm)	49	57	54	52	52
LVDs (mm)	32	35	42	38	36
IVS (mm)	10	9	9	9	9
PW (mm)	10	10	8	8	9
LA (mm)	50	51	43	44	49
LAVI (mL/	92	79	80	Not evaluated	96
E/E′	9.1	8.5	8.2	6.9	7.6
MR severity	Mild-moderate	Mild-moderate	Mild-moderate	Mild-moderate	Mild-moderate
Medication of HF	Titration of bisoprolol for AF rate control		Initiation of enalapril and eplerenone		

Abbreviations: AF, atrial fibrillation; BNP, brain natriuretic peptide; CTRCD, cancer therapy–related cardiac dysfunction; DXR, Doxorubicin; HF, heart failure; IVS, interventricular septum; LA, left atrium; LAVI, left atrial volume index; MR, mitral regurgitation; PW, posterior left ventricular wall.

Table 3
Case 3: acute pericardial effusion after PBSCT

	Pretreatment	Pre-PBSCT (Total DXR 400 mg/m^2)	47 d After PBSCT	3 y After PBSCT
Echocardiogram				
LVEF (%)	67	65	55	53
LVDd (mm)	43	40	43	40
LVDs (mm)	28	24	30	29
IVS (mm)	9	9	10	12
PW (mm)	8	9	11	9
E/A	1.2	1.16	0.80	1.26
DcT	79	175	Not evaluated because of tachycardia	371
E/E'	8.4	8.3	15.9	12.3
Maximum diameter of PE (mm)	None	None	21	None
Other	None	None	Reduced IVC respiratory movement RV and RA collapse (+)	Constrictive pericarditis (−)

Abbreviations: DcT, deceleration time; DXR, Doxorubicin; IVS, interventricular septum; PBSCT, peripheral blood stem cell transplantation; PE, pericardial effusion; PW, posterior left ventricular wall; RA, right atrium; RV, right ventricle.

DISCUSSION

Myocardial dysfunction caused by cardiotoxicity of antineoplastic agents is well known and includes trastuzumab and anthracycline cardiomyopathy as presented here in Cases 1 and 2. Hematopoietic stem cell transplantation (HSCT) can also induce myocardial dysfunction, in addition massive PE because of GVHD as in Case 3.

Case 1 presented acute and re-exacerbated heart failure related to trastuzumab. Cancer therapy–related cardiac dysfunction (CTRCD) manifests in 2% to 27% of patients with cancer treated with trastuzumab,[10,11] and typically occurs during treatment with this drug.[12] Trastuzumab-related cardiomyopathy is usually improved by medical management of heart failure and discontinuing trastuzumab. Rechallenge with trastuzumab is acceptable after improvement in heart failure symptoms and LVEF returning to at least 40%. Even so, trastuzumab-related cardiomyopathy sometimes does not improve completely, with a rate of 20% to 35%.[10,13–15] Furthermore, our case indicates trastuzumab-related cardiomyopathy could re-exacerbate even after complete recovery of cardiac performance. Therefore, heart failure treatment of trastuzumab-related cardiomyopathy should be continued even after the amelioration of cardiac dysfunction as usual heart failure.[16] Over a 10-year follow-up in breast cancer survivors, the cumulative rate of CVD death exceeded that of breast cancer death itself,[6] and ABCDE Steps are recommended for prevention of heart disease: (A) *Awareness* of risks of heart disease and *Aspirin*; (B) *Blood* pressure; (C) *Cholesterol* and *Cigarette* cessation; (D) *Diet* and weight management, *Dose* of chemotherapy or radiation, and *Diabetes* mellitus control; and (E) Exercise and *Echocardiogram.*[17]

Case 2 presented heart failure caused by anthracycline. This was administered to a patient who had undergone recent cardiac surgery and had comorbidities, such as AF, indicating the importance of the presence of comorbidities and early detection of cardiotoxicity. Ewing sarcoma has such a high recurrence rate that VDC/IE-based multimodality adjuvant therapy including anthracycline is recommended.[18] Anthracyclines, such as doxorubicin, mitoxantrone, daunorubicin, and idarubicin, are the key drugs for some solid tumors and hematologic malignancies,[19,20] but they have a risk of adverse cardiac effects, which can be fatal and lead to a poor prognosis for patients with cancer and survivors.[21,22] The incidence of doxorubicin-related cardiac events during chemotherapy increases with cumulative doxorubicin infusion of more than 400 mg/m^2 (5%, 26%, and 48% at cumulative doses of 400, 550, and

650 mg/m^2). However, the cumulative incidence of cardiac dysfunction in long-term follow-up increases even in patients with cumulative doses less than 400 mg/m^2 (9%, 18%, 38%, and 65% at cumulative doses of 250, 350, 450, and 550 mg/m^2).[23] Furthermore, subclinical cardiac dysfunction presented at a rate of about 30% even with low-dose doxorubicin of 180 to 240 mg/m^2.[24] Currently, high-risk patients after the administration of anthracyclines include (1) high-dose anthracycline (eg, doxorubicin $\geq$250 mg/m^2, epirubicin $\geq$600 mg/m^2) and lower-dose anthracyclines (2) with radiation therapy, for which the heart is in the treatment field and regardless of high-dose or lower-dose, (3) with risk factors including age ($\geq$60 years), cardiac dysfunction (eg, borderline LVEF, $\geq$ moderate valvular disease), or multiple cardiac risk factors (eg, smoking, hypertension, diabetes, dyslipidemia, and obesity), or (4) after trastuzumab treatment.[3,25]

The total doxorubicin dose in our case was 345 mg/m^2, indicating a high risk of CTRCD, and open heart surgery may also raise the risk. However, frequent screening by TTE detected early phase CTRCD without symptoms, and LV function was ameliorated by treatment of heart failure. This case demonstrated the importance of detecting subclinical LV dysfunction before a patient presents congestive heart failure. CTRCD caused by anthracyclines is often irreversible, but Cardinale and colleagues[26] revealed it can be reversed if heart failure therapy, such as angiotensin-converting enzyme inhibitor and β-blockers, is administered as soon as possible. Responders have fewer cardiac events, whereas many nonresponders and partial responders experience future cardiac events.[26] To detect early cardiac dysfunction caused by anthracycline, TTE, especially the LVEF and global longitudinal strain, and a troponin assay are recommended at baseline, every 50 mg/m^2 over 240 mg/m^2 administration of anthracycline in terms of doxorubicin, and between 6 and 12 months after completion of therapy.[3,27] In addition, repeated cardiac surveillance is recommended for high-risk survivors.[28]

The recommendation for cardiomyopathy surveillance is presented in **Fig. 1**.

Case 3 shows pericardial cardiotoxicity after HSCT. Pericarditis was caused by idiopathic, viral, bacterial or fungal, neoplastic, autoimmune, or traumatic cause, and accounted for 0.2% of patients hospitalized for CVD. The mortality rate was 1.1% in a general cohort.[29,30] PE developed at a rate of 3.1% to 19% after HSCT, and age (younger children or older adults), stem cell source (especially unrelated donor transplants and cord blood), HLA mismatch, delayed neutrophil engraftment, GVHD prophylaxis (other than cyclosporin A), GVHD, and cytomegalovirus infection have been suggested as risk factors.[31–36] In addition, PE can appear in the late phase.[32,36] Even if PE itself is not fatal, the presence of PE influences the long-term survival rate and treatment-related mortality.[35,36] When PE occurs after HSCT, infection, GVHD and medication, especially calcineurin-inhibitors, such as tacrolimus and cyclosporine, should be considered as a cause. Antibiotics, interruption of calcineurin-inhibitors, or increasing immunosuppressants are advised in such situations with or without pericardiocentesis. In this case, cardiac tamponade caused by GVHD was confirmed. Not only the symptoms of tamponade, but also renal function were ameliorated after pericardiocentesis. Acute renal failure after transplantation is related to poor prognosis and cardiac tamponade often induces renal dysfunction, thus, pericardiocentesis should be considered soon after the appearance of tamponade.[30,37] Not only PE, but also CVD, such as heart failure, coronary disease, and cerebrovascular disease, increase after HSCT, whereas patients after transplantation have increased risk of CVD, such as hypertension, diabetes, and dyslipidemia, which increase the risk of CVD in the long term.[38–41] In addition to baseline CVD risk factors, direct effects, such as chemotherapy and radiation, and indirect effects, such as GVHD and immunosuppressive therapy, cause CVD and de novo CVD risk factors. A model of the relationship between CVD and cancer treatment including HSCT is shown in **Fig. 2**. Long-term observation is necessary for patients after HSCT, in particular those treated with cardiotoxic agents and/or radiation therapy.[38,41]

In addition to the representative cases presented here, clinical heart failure is caused by not only direct myocardial toxicity, but also ischemic cardiomyopathy, valvular disorders, constrictive pericarditis, or right heart failure because of pulmonary hypertension.[42–50] Important cardiotoxicity-related heart failure factors are indicated in **Table 4**. Fluorouracil, a drug commonly used for gastrointestinal cancer, causes myocardial ischemia with a frequency of up to 19%; this sometimes becomes fatal and can induce ischemic cardiomyopathy.[2,45] Radiation therapy affects all structures in the irradiated area, such as pericarditis in an acute manifestation and ischemia, valvular disease, and cardiomyopathy in chronic manifestations.[46,47] BCR-ABL, a tyrosine kinase inhibitor, improves the prognosis of chronic myeloid leukemia dramatically, but dasatinib, a second-generation tyrosine kinase

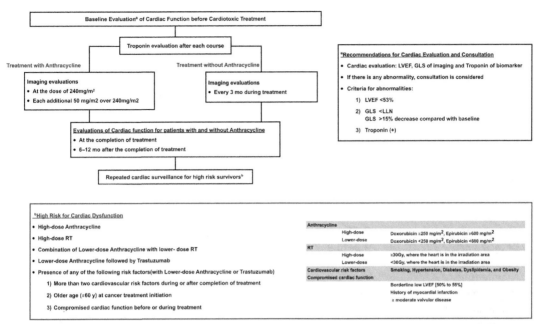

Fig. 1. Surveillance recommendations for early detection of cardiac dysfunction. Baseline evaluation of cardiac function, such as LVEF, GLS, and troponin, is recommended. Troponin after each course and fixed imaging evaluation could detect clinical or subclinical cardiac dysfunction during treatment. No specific evidence for long-term cardiomyopathy surveillance, but repeated evaluation is recommended. GLS, global longitudinal strain; LLN, lower limit of normal; RT, radiation therapy. (*Data from* Refs.[3,27,28])

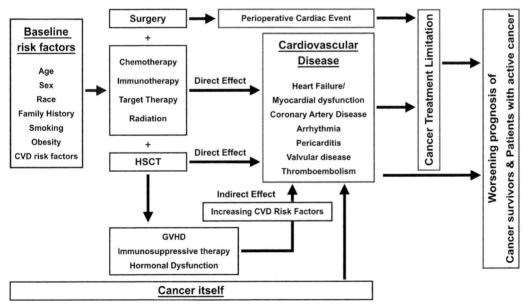

Fig. 2. Model of the relationship between CVD and cancer treatment including HSCT. Many patients with cancer have CVD risk factors at the time of cancer diagnosis. These risk factors affect the cardiotoxicity caused by chemotherapy, immunotherapy, target therapy, radiation, and HSCT itself. In addition, surgery can cause perioperative cardiac events, and HSCT affects cardiotoxicity indirectly including via GVHD, immunosuppressive therapy, and hormonal dysfunction after HSCT. CVD and CVD risk factors worsen the prognosis of cancer survivors and require the cessation or modification of cancer therapy, resulting in a poor prognosis for patients with active cancers. (*Data from* Refs.[5,38,41])

Table 4
Cardiovascular adverse events caused by cancer therapy including left ventricular dysfunction

	CTRCD (%)[a]	CAD	Arrhythmia	VTE	Hypertension	Other
Anthracycline						
Doxorubicin ($\leq$550 mg/m^2)	3–26	–	+/++	?	–	
Epirubicin	0.9–11.4	–		?	–	
Idarubicin	5–18	–	++/+++	?	–	
Alkylating agent						
Cyclophosphamide	7–28	–	–	+	–	
Ifosfamide (>12.5 g/m^2)	17	–	?	?	–	
Antimicrotubule agents						
Docetaxel	2.3–8.0	++	+/++	?	++	
Monoclonal antibodies						
Trastuzumab	2–28	–	++	+/++	++	
Bevacizumab	1.0–10.9	+/++	++	++/+++	++/+++	
Ado-trastuzumab emtansine	1.8	–	++	–	++	
Pertuzumab	0.9–16.0	–	–	–	–	
Small-molecule TKI						
Imatinib	0.3–2.7	+++	–	+	–	
Nilotinib	1	?	++	+	++	PAOD
Dasatinib	8–9	++	++/+++	+/++	++	PAH
Ponatinib	3–15	++	++	++	+++	PAOD
Sunitinib	1–27	++	+	+/++	+++	
Pazopanib	0.6–11.0	+/++	–	++	+++	
Lapatinib	0.9–4.9	–	?	–	–	
Proteasome inhibitors						
Carfilzomib	6.7	+	–	++	+++	
Bortezomib	2.0–7.6	+	++	++	++	
ICI						
Anti-PD-1/PD-L1 monotherapy	0.41	+	++	+	+	Pericardial disease
Anti-CTLA-4 monotherapy	0.07	–	++	+	–	Pericardial disease
Combination ICIs	−1.33	?	++	+	+	Pericardial disease
Miscellaneous						
Tretinoin	1–6	–	–	+	–	
Radiation therapy		+++	–	?	–	Valvular disease Pericardial disease
Without anthracycline	4.4–13.3					
With anthracycline	11.2–32.9					
Stem cell transplantation	5–43	++	++/+++	?	+++	Valvular disease Pericardial disease

Incidence: +++ >10%, ++ 1%–10%, + <1% or rare, ? unknown incidence, and - no recognition.

Abbreviations: CAD, coronary artery disease; ICI, immune checkpoint inhibitor; PAH, pulmonary arterial hypertension; PAOD, peripheral artery occlusive disease; TKI, tyrosine kinase inhibitors; VTE, venous thromboembolism.

[a] CTRCD including myocarditis, noninflammatory ventricular dysfunction.

Data from Refs.[10,41,42,44,47,50]

inhibitor, can induce pulmonary arterial hypertension causing right heart failure.[48] Finally, multiple myeloma itself could provoke cardiac dysfunction because of secondary amyloidosis, and treatment with bortezomib and carfilzomib also cause CTRCD.[49,50] Moreover, immune check-point inhibitor–related myocarditis is drawing attention as an immune-related adverse event. This is rare, but lethal if it becomes fulminant. Conventional heart failure treatment is sometimes insufficient and the administration of high-dose corticosteroid is needed. Steroid pulse and immunosuppressive agents, such as infliximab or mycophenolate, should be considered for patients who have no immediate response to high-dose corticosteroids.[42,43] The adoption of immunotherapy has been expanding, and combination therapy with several immune check-point inhibitors has also been authorized. This will increase the number of patients who develop cardiotoxicity related to immune-related adverse events, and cardiologists need to know how to treat cardiotoxicity caused by immune-related adverse events. Cancer treatment is evolving rapidly and there may be many unknown cancer therapy cardiotoxicities. Therefore, cardiologists and cardio-oncologists must respond to emerging needs regarding cancer therapy–related cardiotoxicities to improve the prognoses of patients with cancer.

SUMMARY

This report summarized the pathophysiology of cancer therapy-related CVD by showing three representative cases. In addition to the classical CTRCD, such as anthracycline cardiomyopathy, new cardiotoxicity has emerged because of cancer treatment showing rapid progression and expansion. It is important for cardiologists and oncologists to understand the pathophysiology of cardiotoxicity following cancer treatment, which potentially improves the overall survival of patients with cancer.

DISCLOSURE

The authors have nothing to disclose.

REFERENCES

1. Quaresma M, Coleman MP, Rachet B. 40-year trends in an index of survival for all cancers combined and survival adjusted for age and sex for each cancer in England and Wales, 1971-2011: a population-based study. Lancet 2015;385(9974): 1206–18.
2. Zamorano JL, Lancellotti P, Rodriguez Muñoz D, et al. 2016 ESC Position Paper on cancer treatments and cardiovascular toxicity developed under the auspices of the ESC Committee for practice guidelines. Eur Heart J 2016;37(36):2768–801.
3. Armenian SH, Lacchetti C, Barac A, et al. Prevention and monitoring of cardiac dysfunction in survivors of adult cancers: American Society of Clinical Oncology clinical practice guideline. J Clin Oncol 2017;35(8):893–911.
4. Reddy P, Shenoy C, Blaes AH. Cardio-oncology in the older adult. J Geriatr Oncol 2017;8(4):308–14.
5. Johnson CB, Davis MK, Law A, et al. Shared risk factors for cardiovascular disease and cancer: implications for preventive health and clinical care in oncology patients. Can J Cardiol 2016;32(7):900–7.
6. Koene RJ, Prizment AE, Blaes A, et al. Shared risk factors in cardiovascular disease and cancer. Circulation 2016;133(11):1104–14.
7. Patnaik JL, Byers T, DiGuiseppi C, et al. Cardiovascular disease competes with breast cancer as the leading cause of death for older females diagnosed with breast cancer: a retrospective cohort study. Breast Cancer Res 2011;13(3):R64.
8. Oeffinger KC, Mertens AC, Sklar CA, et al. Chronic health conditions in adult survivors of childhood cancer. N Engl J Med 2006;355(15):1572–82.
9. Armstrong GT, Kawashima T, Leisenring W, et al. Aging and risk of severe, disabling, life-threatening, and fatal events in the childhood cancer survivor study. J Clin Oncol 2014;32(12):1218–27.
10. Chang HM, Moudgil R, Scarabelli T, et al. Cardiovascular complications of cancer therapy: best practices in diagnosis, prevention, and management: part 1. J Am Coll Cardiol 2017;70(20):2536–51.
11. Slamon Dennis J, Lelyland-Jones B, Shak Steven NL, et al. Use of chemotherapy plus a monoclonal antibody against HER2 for metastatic breast cancer that overexpresses HER2. N Engl J Med 2001;344(11):783–92.
12. De Azambuja E, Procter MJ, Van Veldhuisen DJ, et al. Trastuzumab-associated cardiac events at 8 years of median follow-up in the Herceptin adjuvant trial (BIG 1-01). J Clin Oncol 2014;32(20):2159–65.
13. Suter TM, Procter M, Van Veldhuisen DJ, et al. Trastuzumab-associated cardiac adverse effects in the Herceptin adjuvant trial. J Clin Oncol 2007;25(25): 3859–65.
14. Ewer MS, Vooletich MT, Durand JB, et al. Reversibility of trastuzumab-related cardiotoxicity: new insights based on clinical course and response to medical treatment. J Clin Oncol 2005;23(31): 7820–6.
15. Yoon HJ, Kim KH, Kim JY, et al. Breast cancer chemotherapy-induced left ventricular dysfunction in patients with breast cancer. J Breast Cancer 2016;19(4):402–9.
16. Yancy CW, Jessup M, Bozkurt B, et al. 2013 ACCF/ AHA guideline for the management of heart failure: a

report of the American College of Cardiology Foundation/American Heart Association Task Force on practice guidelines. Circulation 2013;128(16): e240–327.

17. Montazeri K, Unitt C, Foody JM, et al. ABCDE steps to prevent heart disease in breast cancer survivors. Circulation 2014;130(18):157–9.

18. Grier HE, Krailo MD, Tarbell NJ, et al. Addition of ifosfamide and etoposide to standard chemotherapy for Ewing's sarcoma and primitive neuroectodermal tumor of bone. N Engl J Med 2003;348(8): 694–701.

19. Nesbit ME, Gehan EA, Burgert EO, et al. Multimodal therapy for the management of primary, nonmetastatic Ewing's sarcoma of bone: a long-term follow-up of the first intergroup study. J Clin Oncol 1990; 8(10):1664–74.

20. Peters FPJ, Lalisang RI, Fickers MMF, et al. Treatment of elderly patients with intermediate- and high-grade non-Hodgkin's lymphoma: a retrospective population-based study. Ann Hematol 2001; 80(3):155–9.

21. Hershman DL, McBride RB, Eisenberger A, et al. Doxorubicin, cardiac risk factors, and cardiac toxicity in elderly patients with diffuse B-cell non-Hodgkin's lymphoma. J Clin Oncol 2008;26(19): 3159–65.

22. Felker GM, Thompson RE, Hare JM, et al. Underlying causes and long-term survival in patients with initially unexplained cardiomyopathy. N Engl J Med 2000;342(15):1077–84.

23. Swain SM, Whaley FS, Ewer MS. Congestive heart failure in patients treated with doxorubicin: a retrospective analysis of three trials. Cancer 2003; 97(11):2869–79.

24. Vandecruys E, Mondelaers V, de Wolf D, et al. Late cardiotoxicity after low dose of anthracycline therapy for acute lymphoblastic leukemia in childhood. J Cancer Surviv 2012;6(1):95–101.

25. Van Nimwegen FA, Schaapveld M, Janus CPM, et al. Cardiovascular disease after Hodgkin lymphoma treatment: 40-year disease risk. JAMA Intern Med 2015;175(6):1007–17.

26. Cardinale D, Colombo A, Lamantia G, et al. Anthracycline-induced cardiomyopathy. clinical relevance and response to pharmacologic therapy. J Am Coll Cardiol 2010;55(3):213–20.

27. Plana JC, Galderisi M, Barac A, et al. Expert consensus for multimodality imaging evaluation of adult patients during and after cancer therapy: a report from the American Society of Echocardiography and the European Association of Cardiovascular Imaging. J Am Soc Echocardiogr 2014;27(9): 911–39.

28. Armenian SH, Hudson MM, Mulder RL, et al. Recommendations for cardiomyopathy surveillance for survivors of childhood cancer: a report from the International Late Effects of Childhood Cancer Guideline Harmonization Group. Lancet Oncol 2015;16(3):e123–36.

29. Imazio M, Gaita F, LeWinter M. Evaluation and treatment of pericarditis: a systematic review. JAMA 2015;314(14):1498–506.

30. Kytö V, Sipilä J, Rautava P. Clinical profile and influences on outcomes in patients hospitalized for acute pericarditis. Circulation 2014;130(18): 1601–6.

31. Aldoss O, Gruenstein DH, Bass JL, et al. Pericardial effusion after pediatric hematopoietic cell transplant. Pediatr Transplant 2013;17(3):294–9.

32. Liu YC, Chien SH, Fan NW, et al. Risk factors for pericardial effusion in adult patients receiving allogeneic haematopoietic stem cell transplantation. Br J Haematol 2015;169(5):737–45.

33. Versluys AB, Grotenhuis HB, Boelens MJJ, et al. Predictors and outcome of pericardial effusion after hematopoietic stem cell transplantation in children. Pediatr Cardiol 2018;39(2):236–44.

34. Rhodes M, Lautz T, Kavanaugh-Mchugh A, et al. Pericardial effusion and cardiac tamponade in pediatric stem cell transplant recipients. Bone Marrow Transplant 2005;36(2):139–44.

35. Neier M, Jin Z, Kleinman C, et al. Pericardial effusion post-SCT in pediatric recipients with signs and/or symptoms of cardiac disease. Bone Marrow Transplant 2011;46(4):529–38.

36. Chen X, Zou Q, Yin J, et al. Pericardial effusion post transplantation predicts inferior overall survival following allo-hematopoietic stem cell transplant. Bone Marrow Transplant 2016;51(2):303–6.

37. Hahn T, Rondeau C, Shaukat A, et al. Acute renal failure requiring dialysis after allogeneic blood and marrow transplantation identifies very poor prognosis patients. Bone Marrow Transplant 2003;32(4): 405–10.

38. Scott JM, Armenian S, Giralt S, et al. Cardiovascular disease following hematopoietic stem cell transplantation: pathogenesis, detection, and the cardioprotective role of aerobic training. Crit Rev Oncol Hematol 2016;98:222–34.

39. Chow EJ, Mueller BA, Baker KS, et al. Cardiovascular hospitalizations and mortality among recipient of hematopoietic stem cell transplantation. Ann Intern Med 2011;155(1):21–32.

40. Armenian SH, Sun CL, Shannon T, et al. Incidence and predictors of congestive heart failure after autologous hematopoietic cell transplantation. Blood 2011;118(23):6023–9.

41. Armenian SH, Chemaitilly W, Chen M, et al. National Institutes of Health hematopoietic cell transplantation late effects initiative: the Cardiovascular Disease and Associated Risk Factors Working Group report. Biol Blood Marrow Transplant 2017;23(2): 201–10.

42. Lyon AR, Yousaf N, Battisti NML, et al. Immune checkpoint inhibitors and cardiovascular toxicity. Lancet Oncol 2018;19(9):e447–58.

43. Brahmer JR, Lacchetti C, Schneider BJ, et al. Management of immune-related adverse events in patients treated with immune checkpoint inhibitor therapy: American Society of Clinical Oncology Clinical Practice Guideline. J Clin Oncol 2019;36(17): 1714–68.

44. Truong J, Yan AT, Cramarossa G, et al. Chemotherapy-induced cardiotoxicity: detection, prevention, and management. Can J Cardiol 2014;30(8): 869–78.

45. Sara JD, Kaur J, Khodadadi R, et al. 5-fluorouracil and cardiotoxicity: a review. Ther Adv Med Oncol 2018;10. 1758835918780140.

46. Jaworski C, Mariani JA, Wheeler G, et al. Cardiac complications of thoracic irradiation. J Am Coll Cardiol 2013;61(23):2319–28.

47. Van Nimwegen FA, Ntentas G, Darby SC, et al. Risk of heart failure in survivors of Hodgkin lymphoma: effects of cardiac exposure to radiation and anthracyclines. Blood 2017;129(16):2257–65.

48. Pasvolsky O, Leader A, Iakobishvili Z, et al. Tyrosine kinase inhibitor associated vascular toxicity in chronic myeloid leukemia. Cardio Oncol 2015; 1–10. https://doi.org/10.1186/s40959-015-0008-5.

49. Chari A, Stewart AK, Russell SD, et al. Analysis of carfilzomib cardiovascular safety profile across relapsed and/or refractory multiple myeloma clinical trials. Blood Adv 2018;2(13):1633–44.

50. Laubach JP, Moslehi JJ, Francis SA, et al. A retrospective analysis of 3954 patients in phase 2/3 trials of bortezomib for the treatment of multiple myeloma: towards providing a benchmark for the cardiac safety profile of proteasome inhibition in multiple myeloma. Br J Haematol 2017;178(4): 547–60.

Palliative Care in Patients with Advanced Heart Failure

Keisuke Kida, MD, PhD[a],*, Shunichi Doi, MD[b], Norio Suzuki, MD, PhD[c]

KEYWORDS

- Advance care planning • Shared decision making • End-of-life • Opioid • Palliative inotrope
- Hospice

KEY POINTS

- Patients with heart failure (HF) often suffer from total pain; therefore, the support from a multidisciplinary team plays a crucial role to improve quality of life of the patients and their families not only in the terminal phase but also from the early stage.
- In HF, the terms palliative care and terminal care are not synonymous; thus, palliative care should not be initiated from the terminal phase.
- Because HF with fluid retention and low-cardiac output may trigger several unpleasant symptoms, continuous HF treatment is required to alleviate these symptoms in advanced HF.
- Clinicians should fully understand the risks and benefits of outpatient inotropes when they offer these medications to patients with advanced HF.
- Despite its many benefits, hospice care is underused for patients with advanced HF.

INTRODUCTION

Heart failure (HF) is a disease that causes shortness of breath and swelling owing to heart malfunction, which gradually exacerbates and shortens lifespan. The Japanese Circulation Society proposed a clear definition of HF for the general public in 2018.[1] Japan is one of the most rapidly aging societies in the world. It is estimated that by 2025, 30.3% of the total population will be 65 years of age or older and 18.1% of those will be 75 years of age or older.[2] The number of elderly with HF is increasing in this aging population; heart disease, including HF, is the second leading cause of death after cancer. It is reported that one out of every 2 Japanese persons has cancer. The prognosis is improving by early diagnosis and treatment, although the number of deaths is inevitably increasing in the aging society.

Palliative care has been developed as a terminal care for cancer and AIDS; meanwhile, the term "palliative care" is increasingly used with regard to diseases other than cancer, such as life-threatening disease, including cardiovascular and respiratory diseases. The World Health Organization (WHO) promotes the need to prevent and alleviate suffering and improve quality of life (QOL) by early detection of physical and psychosocial distress and appropriate assessment and treatment.

[a] Department of Pharmacology, St. Marianna University School of Medicine, 2-16-1 Sugao Miyamae, Kawasaki, Kanagawa 216-8511, Japan; [b] Division of Cardiology, Department of Internal Medicine, St. Marianna University School of Medicine, 2-16-1 Sugao Miyamae, Kawasaki, Kanagawa 216-8511, Japan; [c] Division of Cardiology, Department of Internal Medicine, St. Marianna University School of Medicine Yokohama City Seibu Hospital, 1197-1 Yasachi-chou, Asahi-ku, Yokohama, Kanagawa 241-0811, Japan
* Corresponding author.
E-mail address: heart-kida@marianna-u.ac.jp

Heart Failure Clin 16 (2020) 243–254
https://doi.org/10.1016/j.hfc.2019.12.006
1551-7136/20/© 2019 Elsevier Inc. All rights reserved.

Patients with HF often suffer from total pain; therefore, the support from a multidisciplinary team plays a crucial role in improving QOL of patients and their families not only in the terminal phase but also from the early stage. Various medical devices have contributed to better prognosis. In the terminal phase, QOL is the most important factor, and deactivation of the medical device should also be considered for providing better QOL. One of the goals of palliative care is to assist complex decision making. According to the WHO report in 2014,[3] cardiovascular disease accounts for approximately 40% of the diseases requiring palliative care, although this fact has not been fully recognized in Japan. In 2016, the Ministry of Health, Labor, and Welfare in Japan finally announced a policy to develop a medical care system for palliative care of cardiovascular disease; more education for medical workers is thus called for in palliative care for HF.[4]

Advance Care Planning and Shared Decision Making in Heart Failure

It is no longer appropriate to assume that palliative care should be initiated only as a last resort when traditional HF management fails to fulfill a patient's goal.[5] It can often be difficult to determine the timing of palliative care referral; therefore, it is indispensable to provide advance care planning (ACP) for future changes in conditions, including the end of life.

ACP refers to the entire process in which the health care professionals share the treatment and lifestyle desired by a patient and his or her family in advance before his or her decision-making ability declines. ACP aims to fulfill one's life on his or her own when death is approaching. Palliative care, and ACP as well, should be initiated from the early stage when HF becomes symptomatic. The physical, psychological, and mental needs of patients should be frequently evaluated by a multidisciplinary team.

One review provides the evidence from the 13 randomized controlled trials and suggests that interventions that involve patients to change clinical practice, reminder systems, and educational meetings have the greatest effect in improving the implementation of ACP in HF.[6] The key messages of this review are shown in **Box 1**.

In 2010, the Japanese Circulation Society published "Statement for end-stage cardiovascular care" and defined the following 4 items as an end-stage HF status[7]:

1. Even though the patients are appropriately treated,
2. Those complain of chronic HF symptoms and frequently require intravenous drug therapy.

Box 1
Key messages of advance care planning in heart failure

Key messages

What is already known on this subject?

- Advance care planning (ACP) is widely advocated to provide better care at the end of life for patients suffering from heart failure.
- However, clinicians appear hesitant to engage with ACP.
- Interventions to better engage patients with ACP have been evaluated. However, a systematic review and metaanalysis of clinician-targeted interventions are missing.

What might this study add?

- Clinician-targeted interventions can help health care professionals to engage with ACP for patients suffering from heart failure.
- Interventions that involve patients to change clinicians' practice, reminder systems, and educational meetings seem to be among the most effective approaches to facilitate ACP.
- This effect was observed especially when the intervention simultaneously enabled both clinicians and patients to engage with ACP.

How might this impact on clinical practice?

- Interventions that enable clinicians to engage with ACP in heart failure need to be developed.
- Given the constraints of clinical practice, barriers and facilitators for such a complex intervention need to be identified.
- Patients with heart failure hold a key to change clinical practice and need to be enabled to engage clinicians with ACP.

From Schichtel M, Wee B, Perera R, et al. Clinician-targeted interventions to improve advance care planning in heart failure: a systematic review and meta-analysis. Heart 2019; 105:1316–24; with permission. (Key messages in original).

---

3. Their hospitalization histories account for once or more in 6 months and those with low left ventricular ejection fraction.
4. Those are diagnosed that the terminal phase is getting close.

The premise of this statement is that an appropriate treatment of HF is provided. Unlike advanced cancer in which an aggressive treatment is not performed at the terminal phase, HF requires continuous treatment until it alleviates its symptoms. In HF, the terms palliative and terminal care are not

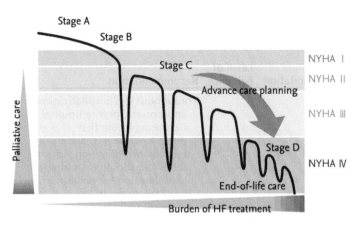

Fig. 1. Palliative and end-of-life care in the time course of HF. (*From* Okumura T, Sawamura A, Murohara T. Palliative and end-of-life care for heart failure patients in an aging society. Korean J Intern Med 2018;33(6):1042; with permission.)

synonymous; thus, palliative care should not be initiated from the terminal phase (**Fig. 1**).[8]

Palliative care for HF includes 4 principles, although principles 2, 3, and 4 are actually often neglected:

1. Alleviation of physical pain and basic symptoms according to the guidelines
2. Mental care through supportive communication
3. ACP
4. Support for decision making concerning principles 1, 2, and 3

Palliative and hospice care remain grossly underused for HF because of both general and disease-specific barriers.[9] It has been described that there is a pressing need to integrate palliative care into conventional care for patients with HF. Clinicians, researchers, and policymakers should set an agenda for available health care services to the needs of patients and their families. It seems that the time has come for medical culture to accept the importance of the patients' values, goals, and preferences in guiding medical

decisions.[10] The HF guidelines are changing to include language around shared decision making for major procedures and *end-of-life* care.[11] However, although the cultural norms seem to be moving in this direction, the science regarding how to best deliver patient-centered care (basic, clinical, delivery, and policy) is still developing (**Fig. 2**).[12]

Heart Failure End of Life

The recommendations of palliative care in the HF guidelines are shown in **Table 1**.[8] The current review discusses the integration of guidelines and evidence-based palliative care into HF end-of-life care.[13] The North American and European HF Societies recommend the integration of palliative care into the HF programs. ACP, shared decision making, a routine measurement of symptoms and QOL, and specialist palliative care at HF end of life are identified as key components to an effective HF palliative care program. There is limited evidence to support the effectiveness of the individual elements. However, results from the palliative care in HF trial suggest that an integrated HF palliative

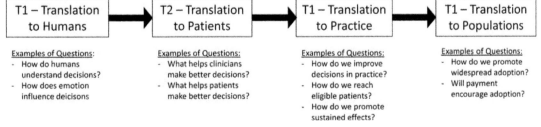

Fig. 2. The science of decision making in advanced HF using a translational science framework. There are 2 important lessons from a survey of the science of decision making in advanced HF. The first lesson from the overview is that it is not linear. Although it would make sense for the formative T1 work to occur before the T4 work, this is not the reality. The second lesson from the discussion is the increasing societal demand and a changing norm around the importance of patient involvement and patient-centered care. (*From* Matlock DD, McGuire WC, Magid M, et al. Decision making in advanced heart failure: bench, bedside, practice, and policy. Heart Fail Rev. 2017;22(5):560; with permission.)

Table 1
Recommended palliative care described in the heart failure guidelines

	Class of Recommendation	Level of Evidence	Recommendation
2013 ACCF/AHA Guideline for the Management of Heart Failure	Class I	B	Throughout the hospitalization as appropriate, before hospital discharge, at the first postdischarge visit, and in subsequent follow-up visits, the following should be addressed: consideration for palliative care or hospice care in selected patients
	Class I	B	Palliative and supportive care is effective for patients with symptomatic advanced HF to improve QOL
The 2013 International Society for Heart and Lung Transplantation Guidelines for mechanical circulatory support: executive summary	Class IIa	C	Palliative care consultation should be a component of the treatment of end-stage HF during the evaluation phase for MCS. In addition, management, goals, and preferences to symptoms for end of life should be discussed with patients receiving MCS as DT
	Class I	C	Consultation with palliative medicine should be considered before MCS device implantation to facilitate discussion of end-of-life issues and establish an advance directive or living will, particularly when implanted as DT
2016 ESC Guidelines for the Diagnosis and Treatment of Acute and Chronic Heart Failure	Class I	A	It is recommended that patients with HF are enrolled in a multidisciplinary care management program to reduce the risk of HF hospitalization and mortality
Guidelines for Acute and Chronic Heart Failure (JCS 2017/JHFS 2017)	Class I	B	Perform advanced care planning, which is the process of dialogue about medical treatment with patients and families in advance before the ability of decision making is failed
	Class I	C	Continue treatment of HF and complications and aim for palliation of coexisting symptoms
	Class II	C	Frequent assessment of physical, psychological, and spiritual needs of patients by multidisciplinary team

Abbreviations: ACCF, American College of Cardiology Foundation; AHA, American Heart Association; DT, destination therapy; ESC, European Society of Cardiology; JCS, Japanese Circulation Society; JHFS, Japanese Heart Failure Society; MCS, mechanical circulatory support.

From Okumura T, Sawamura A, Murohara T. Palliative and end-of-life care for heart failure patients in an aging society. Korean J Intern Med 2018;33(6):1041; with permission.

care program can significantly improve QOL of patients with HF at end of life. Integrating a palliative approach to HF end-of-life care helps to ensure patients receive the care that is congruent with their values, wishes, and preferences. Specialist palliative care referrals are limited to patients with HF who are truly at end of life.

Management and Symptoms with Advanced Heart Failure

The main symptoms in terminal HF are dyspnea, general fatigue, pain, loss of appetite, and depression. It has been reported that, of the patients with terminal HF, 60% to 88% reveal dyspnea; 69% to 82% have general fatigue, and 35% to 78% suffer from pain.[14–16] The questionnaire assessed the symptoms requiring palliative care for patients with HF in Japan.[17] Dyspnea (91%) was the most common symptom, followed by anxiety (71%), depression (61%), and malaise (57%), whereas pain (34%) and leg edema (29%) were relatively rare.

In addition, mental health problems, such as depression, anxiety, and sleeplessness, are often identified in these patients; it is presumed that 70% of the patients with terminal HF are hospitalized for depression.[18] Because HF with fluid retention and low-cardiac output may trigger these symptoms, it is required to alleviate the following symptoms in continuous HF treatment of advanced HF.

Dyspnea
Dyspnea is the most frequent symptom in terminal HF. Diuretics and vasodilators are used to improve the cause of pulmonary congestion; however, this medication method has many difficulties in alleviating symptoms because of various factors, such as lower blood pressure and renal dysfunction. The efficacy and safety of small amounts of opioids,

including morphine, on treatment-resistant dyspnea have been reported.[19,20] The effect of opioid treatment on not only dyspnea but also pain and anxiety has been recognized, particularly in palliative care for the patients with tachypnea. Meanwhile, side effects, such as nausea, vomiting, and constipation, and overdose in the elderly and patients with renal dysfunction require full attention. Respiratory depression is a rare but possible side effect; thus, terminally ill patients with unstable respiratory conditions should be carefully observed for changes in respiratory frequency and patterns. Based on the findings, Ohmori and colleagues[21] have succeeded in relieving refractory dyspnea without adverse events and establishing a protocol concerning the use of morphine hydrochloride in patients with HF with renal insufficiency (**Table 2**). The use of opioids in patients with HF with renal insufficiency is a great concern. Therefore, further studies are called for. The administration of benzodiazepines is generally considered in patients with mental factors and strong anxiety, although the effect of benzodiazepines is limited compared with that of opioids.

Pain
The higher the prevalence of pain, the more severe the New York Heart Association (NYHA) cardiac function classification.[22] The trigger of pain is considered because of HF itself, comorbidities, and mental stress, although it often can be difficult to identify the major trigger. Several analgesic agents that are developed primarily for conditions other than pain and with various biologic sites of action are available (**Table 3**). These analgesic agents include nonsteroidal anti-inflammatory drugs (NSAIDs), antidepressant agents, and antiepileptic drugs.[23] NSAID use should be avoided as much as possible because the use of NSAIDs

Table 2
Protocol of morphine hydrochloride usage for patients with HF with renal impairment

GFR (mL/min)	Initial Dose (mg/h)	Background Infusion (mg/h)	Criteria for Increasing Background Infusion	Criteria for Decreasing or Interrupting Background Infusion	Bolus Dose	Bolus Interval (min)
15–30 −15	0.5	0–1 0–0.5	Need for 3 or more boli in 2 consecutive hours	RR <12, RASS < −1 and any other adverse events	Same as 1 h amount setting	30

Abbreviations: GFR, glomerular filtration rate; RASS, Richmond Agitation-Sedation Scale; RR, respiratory rate.
From Ohmori T, Mizuno A, Kawai F, et al. Morphine use for heart failure patients with renal insufficiency. J Palliat Med. 2019;22(6):617-8; with permission.

Table 3
Nonopioid analgesic agents for acute and chronic pain

Drug[a]	Dose[b]	Indication	Side Effects and Risks[c]	Other Information
Acetamin-ophen	650 mg orally every 4–6 h; maximum dose, 4000 mg/d; also available as injection	Mild to moderate pain	Overdose can cause liver damage	No evidence of an effect on neuropathic pain
Aspirin	350–650 mg orally every 4 h; maximum dose, 3600 mg/d; individual doses for rheumatic diseases	Mild pain (temporary use), inflammatory rheumatic diseases	Nausea, dyspepsia, abdominal pain, bleeding tendency, tinnitus, headache, dizziness, insomnia, hypersensitivity reactions, risk of gastrointestinal bleeding	Contraindicated in patients with known hypersensitivity; should not be used in children under 16 y of age (risk of Reye syndrome), no evidence of an effect on neuropathic pain
NSAIDs	Dose depends on the specific drug	Mild to moderate pain, pain associated with inflammation	Nausea, dyspepsia, diarrhea, constipation, headache, dizziness, somnolence, hypersensitivity reactions; risks of gastrointes-tinal bleeding, myocardial infarction, stroke	Contraindicated in patients with known hypersensitivity, recommended dose is the lowest effective dose for the shortest period; no evidence of an effect on neuropathic pain
Amitripty-line[d]	25–150 mg orally once daily or in 2 divided doses[e]; maximum single dose, 75 mg; daily doses >75 mg/d should be used with caution in patients >65 y of age	Neuropathic pain (first-line therapy), fibromyalgia, prevention of tension-type headache or migraine	Somnolence, tremor, dizziness, headache, drowsiness, tachycardia, orthostatic hypotension, dry mouth, constipation, nausea, micturition disorder, weight gain, hyperhidrosis, decreased libido, increased risk of suicidal thoughts	Patients with poor metabolism of CYP2D6 require lower doses, abrupt discontinuation should be avoided, contraindicated in patients with recent myocardial infarction or cardiac rhythm disorders, caution required if used with other serotonergic agents
Duloxetine	60–120 mg orally once daily or in 2 divided doses[e]	Neuropathic pain (first-line therapy), chronic musculoskeletal pain, fibromyalgia	Nausea, headache, dry mouth, somnolence, dizziness, increased blood pressure, increased risk of suicidal thoughts	Abrupt discontinuation should be avoided, caution required if used with other serotonergic agents

(continued on next page)

Table 3
(continued)

Drug[a]	Dose[b]	Indication	Side Effects and Risks[c]	Other Information
Gabapentin	900–3600 mg/d orally in 3 divided doses[e]	First-line therapy for neuropathic pain	Dizziness, somnolence, peripheral edema, fever, infection, nausea, lack of coordination, blurred vision, increased risk of suicidal thoughts	Dose adjustment required in patients with compromised renal function; misuse, abuse, and dependence have been reported
Pregabalin	300–600 mg/d orally in 2 divided doses[e]	Neuropathic pain (first-line therapy), fibromyalgia	Dizziness, somnolence, headache, peripheral edema, nausea, weight gain, disorientation, blurred vision, increased risk of suicidal thoughts	Dose adjustment required in patients with compromised renal function; misuse, abuse, and dependence have been reported
Lidocaine, 1.8% or 5% patch	1–3 patches applied to intact skin for up to 12 h/d	Peripheral neuropathic pain	Application-site pain, pruritus, erythema, and skin irritation	Approved by FDA and EMA for postherpetic neuralgia only
Capsaicin, 8% patch	1–4 patches applied to intact skin for 30 or 60 min every 3 mo	Peripheral neuropathic pain	Application-site pain and erythema, transient increase in blood pressure, risk of reduced sensation	Applied by a health care professional wearing nitrile gloves

Abbreviations: CYP2D6, denotes cytochrome P-450 2D6; EMA, European Medicines Agency; FDA, Food and Drug Administration.

[a] The drugs listed are those commonly used, but the list does not include all analgesics used for all pain conditions.
[b] Doses are given for adults.
[c] For a comprehensive list of side effects, risks, contraindications, and warnings, refer to the product information for each drug.
[d] Other tricyclic antidepressants (imipramine, desipramine, and nortriptyline) have not been evaluated as extensively for the treatment of pain but may be associated with more acceptable side-effect profiles.
[e] The starting dose is lower.
From Finnerup NB. Nonnarcotic methods of pain management. N Engl J Med. 2019;380(25):2440–8; with permission.

has a risk of worsening renal dysfunction and fluid retention in patients with terminal HF. Acetaminophen is recommended as a nonnarcotic analgesic; when pain is not well controlled by using acetaminophen, an additional administration of opioids should be considered.

General fatigue
Before the initiation of therapeutic intervention for general fatigue, it is indispensable to identify low-cardiac output and the presence or absence of depression, hypothyroidism, anemia, excessive administration of diuretics, abnormal electrolyte, sleep apnea, and latent infection. Fatigue owing to HF is often unresponsive to drug therapy; thus, non–drug treatment, such as aerobic exercise and energy-sparing therapy, might be effective.[24]

Depression/anxiety
Depression in patients with HF is a factor for poor prognosis and is associated with decreased QOL.[25] In general, selective serotonin reuptake inhibitors (SSRIs), serotonin noradrenaline reuptake inhibitors, and noradrenaline serotonergic antidepressants are selected. Since the increased mortality has been currently reported by the coadministration of beta-blockers and SSRIs, the optimal antidepressant in patients with HF has not been established yet.[26] It has also been

demonstrated that the use of antidepressants does not necessarily improve the prognosis in patients with HF.[27–29] Tricyclic antidepressants should be used cautiously in patients with HF because they increase the risk of side effects in the cardiovascular system, such as QT prolongation and anticholinergic action. Benzodiazepines are the first choice for anxiety; when depression is present, the administration of antidepressant medications is also considered. In addition, nonpharmacologic therapy, including exercise therapy, cardiac rehabilitation provided by a multidisciplinary team as a comprehensive program, and counseling by a mental specialist, is also effective.[30,31]

Delirium

Delirium is frequently observed in patients with terminal HF, particularly in elderly patients, because low-cardiac output greatly affects delirium. It is vital to distinguish dementia from depression and to intervene at an early stage to prevent the exacerbation of delirium. In dementia and depression, the symptoms are relatively stable, whereas typical delirium is characterized by its exacerbation at night. A heart team should regularly evaluate the environment and drugs (antihypertensive drugs, beta-blockers, antiarrhythmic drugs, dopamine agonists, sympathomimetics, anticholinergic drugs, sleep drugs, and antianxiety drugs) that may cause or worsen delirium to ensure its safety. In severe cases, consultation by a psychiatrist and prescription of antipsychotic drugs should be considered.

End-stage pain

The use of an adequate amount of sedation is a last resort to reduce the level of consciousness in terminal patients with HF with distress to alleviate suffering. Midazolam is the benzodiazepine most frequently used for procedural sedation; the desired effect is found by titration until desired effect is achieved. Hamatani and colleagues[32] reported that dexmedetomidine and midazolam were commonly used for palliative sedation in terminally ill patients with HF in Japan. The Richmond Agitation-Sedation Scale was significantly reduced after treatment in both the dexmedetomidine and the midazolam groups. Since blood pressure and heart rate were not changed after the administration of both drugs at maximum dose, which suggested that the feasibility of these drugs should be limited only in the selected terminally ill patients with HF.

The SPICE III trial was an investigation for a light sedation strategy in the real world. Among the 4000 trial patients, that reality translated into a limited ability to deliver a protocol-defined level of light sedation within 24 hours after study inclusion or during the first 2 full days after randomization. The clinicians selected deep sedation in more than half of the patients. Nearly 75% patients in the dexmedetomidine group received propofol, benzodiazepines, or both at lower doses than the patients assigned to receive usual care. The duration of sedative administration was similar in the 2 groups. The trial's primary outcome of 90-day mortality presupposed that differences in pharmacologic management and adherence to the protocol directives of light sedation in the 2 groups would result in improved outcomes in the dexmedetomidine group. Unfortunately, the similarity in administered sedatives and the frequency of deep sedation in the 2 groups make it challenging to interpret the primary finding that there were no between-group differences in the rate of death at 90 days or in other secondary outcomes.[33] The SPICE III trial should be viewed as a call to study clinical decision making because it pertains to depth of sedation and pharmacologic choices. Understanding these management methods could enhance trial design and analysis and heighten insight into improving clinical practice. Deep sedation immobilizes patients, limits communication, increases costs and mortality, and reduces the likelihood of meaningful recovery. Understanding the differences in how sedation should be administered and what drives these variations is essential in providing improved care. Other areas worthy of investigation include pharmacokinetic and pharmacogenomics guidance, based on age, as noted in the SPICE III trial, but also on sex and other characteristics, on personalizing sedative choices for patients and on assessing the relationship between sedatives and restorative sleep.[34]

Prevention of opioid overdose

In theory, all patients who are treated with opioids incur a risk of overdose. However, several factors increase that risk, including sleep-disordered breathing, end-organ dysfunction leading to impaired medication clearance, pulmonary disease, and concomitant use of sedating medications.[35] The number and severity of risk factors should remain within the beneficial range, and the benefits of prescription opioids must outweigh the risk of overdose. The revised Risk Index for Overdose or Severe Opioid-Induced Respiratory Depression (RIOSORD) is a validated instrument used to estimate the risk of overdose in opioid-treated patients.[36,37] The predicted probability of opioid-induced respiratory depression within 6 months after initiation ranges from 1.9% in the lowest-risk group to 83.4% in the highest-risk group. According to the RIOSORD, it should be noted that HF is classified into risk class 2 at 7 points for positive response.

Palliative inotrope therapy

The role of palliative inotropes is changing in tandem with advances in chronic HF care. However, there remains a profound lack of data and guidance on the effect of palliative inotropes on QOL and mortality and little consensus on how this therapy can be optimally used in contemporary practice. Chuzi and colleagues[38] provided a framework for the prescription and management of palliative inotropes, including a discussion of potential risks and benefits and a roadmap for how to initiate, maintain, and wean them.

There are several important findings from this systematic review. First, the quality of data assessing the risks and benefits of ambulatory intravenous inotropes, even among randomized controlled trials, is limited, which warrants careful consideration when interpreting results. Second, most studies are small; thus, the estimates are plagued by wide confidence intervals. Third, the data for inotropes as palliative therapy are particularly lacking, which limits the ability to summarize comparative risks and benefits in most patients with advanced HF who are not eligible for mechanical circulatory support or transplantation. However, based on the available evidence, inotrope infusions seem to improve NYHA functional class. The limited evidence suggests that inotropes should not increase the risk of death. Although hospitalizations and ventricular arrhythmias are common, the above-mentioned evidence is insufficient to conclude whether inotropes affect the

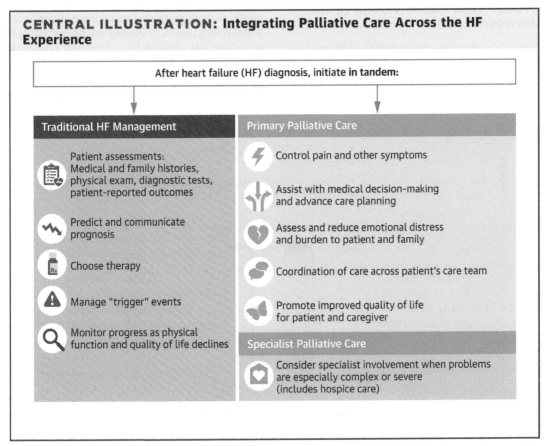

CENTRAL ILLUSTRATION: Integrating Palliative Care Across the HF Experience

After heart failure (HF) diagnosis, initiate **in tandem:**

Traditional HF Management

- Patient assessments: Medical and family histories, physical exam, diagnostic tests, patient-reported outcomes
- Predict and communicate prognosis
- Choose therapy
- Manage "trigger" events
- Monitor progress as physical function and quality of life declines

Primary Palliative Care

- Control pain and other symptoms
- Assist with medical decision-making and advance care planning
- Assess and reduce emotional distress and burden to patient and family
- Coordination of care across patient's care team
- Promote improved quality of life for patient and caregiver

Specialist Palliative Care

- Consider specialist involvement when problems are especially complex or severe (includes hospice care)

Fig. 3. Integrating palliative care across the HF experience. Core domains of primary palliative care (eg, symptom assessment and management, psychosocial support, ACP) may be seamlessly integrated within usual HF disease and device management. When appropriate, specialty palliative care services may be initiated to address complex or intractable palliative needs. The timing of these referrals should be based on patient need, not prognosis, and can be initiated at any point during the HF trajectory. Given that symptoms, functional status, and QOL are not perfectly correlated, it is important that palliative needs such as symptoms and QOL be routinely and systematically monitored throughout the patient's HF care trajectory. (*From* Kavalieratos, Gelfman LP, Tycon LE, et al. Palliative care in heart failure: rationale, evidence, and future priorities. JACC 2017;70(15):1921; with permission.)

risk of these events. Finally, outpatient inotrope infusions are relatively expensive, whereas it seems to be cost-saving compared with ongoing hospitalization in a bridge-to-transplant population, and it is unclear whether they are cost-effective as palliative therapy.[39]

It is important for clinicians to understand the risks and benefits of outpatient inotropes when offering them to patients with advanced HF. Inotrope infusions improve NYHA functional class, but their impact on heart rate, their impact on QOL, and the risks of hospitalization and ventricular arrhythmia are unclear. This review provides a summary of the available evidence on the risks and benefits of outpatient inotropes, which can be used to more effectively counsel patients and families considering inotropes as a treatment option.

IMPORTANCE OF MULTIDISCIPLINARY TEAM APPROACH FOR PALLIATIVE, END OF LIFE, AND HOSPICE CARE

Particularly given the unpredictable trajectory of HF, waiting for a "trigger" event at which to initiate a palliative approach, either primary palliative care or specialty palliative care consultation,

perpetuates the false dichotomy of palliative versus (rather than palliative plus) life-prolonging therapy. In fact, there are often multiple natural opportunities to consider integrating various palliative domains throughout the HF trajectory (**Fig. 3**).[5] One nationwide cross-sectional questionnaire survey indicated the possible associations between palliative care conferences and positive outcomes when performing palliative care for patients with terminal patients with HF in Japan.[40]

Hospice care is team-based palliative care typically reserved for the patients with a life expectancy of 6 months or less. It can be provided to any patient with a life-limiting illness and combines medical care, pain management, and emotional and spiritual support. Although palliative care may be received alongside disease-directed treatment, hospice care focuses on comfort and QOL when a cure is no longer possible. It is a model for high-quality patient-centered care for the patients facing a life-limiting illness.[41] Despite the benefits of hospice care, the patients face significant barriers to receiving timely referrals to that care stemming from the unique course of HF, and the difficulty there is in providing an accurate prognosis (**Fig. 4**).

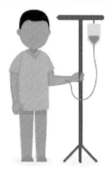

Disease Factors
- Unpredictable trajectory
- Symptom burden
- Frequent exacerbations
- Need for invasive palliative therapies

Policy Factors
- 6-mo survival requirement
- Low fixed daily payment rate
- No concurrent care option

Clinical Factors
- Difficult prognostication
- Discomfort with palliative care
- Lack of training in heart failure for hospice staff

Other Factors
- Patients overestimate survival
- Lack of research in palliative care in heart failure
- Lack of integration of palliative care with cardiology

Fig. 4. Barriers to hospice use in patients with HF. (*From* Cross SH, Kamal AH, Taylor DH Jr, et al. Hospice use among patients with heart failure. Card Fail Rev. 2019;5(2):93–8; with permission.)

SUMMARY

In HF, the terms palliative and terminal care are not synonymous; thus, palliative care should not be initiated from the terminal phase. Because HF with fluid retention and low-cardiac output may trigger several unpleasant symptoms, continuous HF treatment is required to alleviate these symptoms in advanced HF. The patients with HF often suffer from total pain; therefore, the support from a multidisciplinary team plays a crucial role in improving QOL of the patients and their families not only in the terminal phase but also from the early stage.

DISCLOSURE

The authors have nothing to disclose.

REFERENCES

1. Tsutsui H, et al. Guidelines for diagnosis and treatment of acute and chronic heart failure (JCS 2017/JHFS 2017). Available at: http://www.jcirc.or.jp/guideline/pdf/JCS2017_tsutsui_h.pdf. Accessed August 23, 2019. [Article in Japanese].

2. Available at: https://www.mhlw.go.jp/seisakunitsuite/bunya/hukushi_kaigo/kaigo_koureisha/chiiki-houkatsu/dl/link1-1.pdf [Article in Japanese]. Accessed August 23, 2019.

3. WHO Global Atlas on Palliative Care at the End of Life. Available at: https://www.who.int/nmh/Global_Atlas_of_Palliative_Care.pdf. Accessed August 23, 2019.

4. Available at: https://www.mhlw.go.jp/file/05-Shingikai-10901000-Kenkoukyoku-Soumuka/0000185125.pdf [Article in Japanese]. Accessed August 23, 2019.

5. Kavalieratos D, Gelfman LP, Tycon LE, et al. Palliative care in heart failure: rationale, evidence, and future priorities. J Am Coll Cardiol 2017;70:1919–30.

6. Schichtel M, Wee B, Perera R, et al. Clinician-targeted interventions to improve advance care planning in heart failure: a systematic review and meta-analysis. Heart 2019;105(17):1316–24.

7. Nonogi H, et al. Statement for end-stage cardiovascular care (JCS 2010). Available at: http://www.j-circ.or.jp/guideline/pdf/JCS2010_nonogi_h.pdf [Article in Japanese]. Accessed August 23, 2019.

8. Okumura T, Sawamura A, Murohara T. Palliative and end-of-life care for heart failure patients in an aging society. Korean J Intern Med 2018;33:1039–49.

9. Warraich HJ, Meier DE. Serious-illness care 2.0: meeting the needs of patients with heart failure. N Engl J Med 2019;380(26):2492–4.

10. Barry MJ, Edgman-Levitan S. Shared decision making–the pinnacle of patient-centered care. N Engl J Med 2012;366:780–1.

11. Yancy CW, Jessup M, Bozkurt B, et al. 2013 ACCF/AHA guideline for the management of heart failure: a report of the American College of Cardiology Foundation/American Heart Association Task Force on practice guidelines. J Am Coll Cardiol 2013;62:e147–239.

12. Matlock DD, McGuire WC, Magid M, et al. Decision making in advanced heart failure: bench, bedside, practice, and policy. Heart Fail Rev 2017;22(5):559–64.

13. Maciver J, Ross HJ. A palliative approach for heart failure end-of-life care. Curr Opin Cardiol 2018;33(2):202–7.

14. Krumholz HM, Phillips RS, Hamel MB, et al. Resuscitation preferences among patients with severe congestive heart failure: results from the SUPPORT project. Study to understand prognoses and preferences for outcomes and risks of treatments. Circulation 1998;98:648–55.

15. Levenson JW, McCarthy EP, Lynn J, et al. The last six months of life for patients with congestive heart failure. J Am Geriatr Soc 2000;48:S101–9.

16. Solano JP, Gomes B, Higginson IJ. A comparison of symptom prevalence in far advanced cancer, AIDS, heart disease, chronic obstructive pulmonary disease and renal disease. J Pain Symptom Manage 2006;31:58–69.

17. Kuragaichi T, Kurozumi Y, Ohishi S, et al. Nationwide survey of palliative care for patients with heart failure in Japan. Circ J 2018;82(5):1336–43.

18. Rutledge T, Reis VA, Linke SE, et al. Depression in heart failure a meta-analytic review of prevalence, intervention effects, and associations with clinical outcomes. J Am Coll Cardiol 2006;48:1527–37.

19. Johnson MJ, McDonagh TA, Harkness A, et al. Morphine for the relief of breathlessness in patients with chronic heart failure–a pilot study. Eur J Heart Fail 2002;4:753–6.

20. Williams SG, Wright DJ, Marshall P, et al. Safety and potential benefits of low dose diamorphine during exercise in patients with chronic heart failure. Heart 2003;89:1085–6.

21. Ohmori T, Mizuno A, Kawai F, et al. Morphine use for heart failure patients with renal insufficiency. J Palliat Med 2019;22(6):617–8.

22. Evangelista LS, Sackett E, Dracup K. Pain and heart failure: unrecognized and untreated. Eur J Cardiovasc Nurs 2009;8:169–73.

23. Finnerup NB. Nonnarcotic methods of pain management. N Engl J Med 2019;380(25):2440–8.

24. Schaefer KM, Shober Potylycki MJ. Fatigue associated with congestive heart failure: use of Levine's conservation model. J Adv Nurs 1993;18:260–8.

25. Sherwood A, Blumenthal JA, Trivedi R, et al. Relationship of depression to death or hospitalization in patients with heart failure. Arch Intern Med 2007;167:367–73.

26. Fosbøl EL, Gislason GH, Poulsen HE, et al. Prognosis in heart failure and the value of β-blockers are altered by the use of antidepressants and depend on the type of antidepressants used. Circ Heart Fail 2009;2:582–90.

27. O'Connor CM, Jiang W, Kuchibhatla M, et al. SADHART-CHF Investigators. Safety and efficacy of sertraline for depression in patients with heart failure: results of the SADHART-CHF (Sertraline Against Depression and Heart Disease in Chronic Heart Failure) trial. J Am Coll Cardiol 2010;56:692–9.

28. May HT, Horne BD, Carlquist JF, et al. Depression after coronary artery disease is associated with heart failure. J Am Coll Cardiol 2009;53:1440–7.

29. Angermann CE, Gelbrich G, Störk S, et al, MOOD-HF Study Investigators and Committee Members. Effect of escitalopram on all-cause mortality and hospitalization in patients with heart failure and depression: the MOOD-HF randomized clinical trial. JAMA 2016;315:2683–93.

30. Milani RV, Lavie CJ. Impact of cardiac rehabilitation on depression and its associated mortality. Am J Med 2007;120:799–806.

31. Tu RH, Zeng ZY, Zhong GQ, et al. Effects of exercise training on depression in patients with heart failure: a systematic review and meta-analysis of randomized controlled trials. Eur J Heart Fail 2014;16:749–57.

32. Hamatani Y, Nakai E, Nakamura E, et al. Survey of palliative sedation at end of life in terminally ill heart failure patients–a single-center experience of 5-year follow-up. Circ J 2019;83(7):1607–11.

33. Shehabi Y, Howe BD, Bellomo R, et al. Early sedation with dexmedetomidine in critically ill patients. N Engl J Med 2019;380(26):2506–17.

34. Coursin DB, Skrobik Y. What is safe sedation in the ICU? N Engl J Med 2019;380(26):2577–8.

35. Babu KM, Brent J, Juurlink DN. Prevention of opioid overdose. N Engl J Med 2019;380(23):2246–55.

36. Zedler BK, Saunders WB, Joyce AR, et al. Validation of a screening risk index for serious prescription opioid-induced respiratory depression or overdose in a US commercial health plan claims database. Pain Med 2018;19:68–78.

37. Zedler B, Xie L, Wang L, et al. Development of a risk index for serious prescription opioid-induced respiratory depression or overdose in Veterans' Health Administration patients. Pain Med 2015;16:1566–79.

38. Chuzi S, Allen LA, Dunlay SM, et al. Palliative inotrope therapy: a narrative review. JAMA Cardiol 2019. https://doi.org/10.1001/jamacardio.2019.2081.

39. Nizamic T, Murad MH, Allen LA, et al. Ambulatory inotrope infusions in advanced heart failure. A systematic review and meta-analysis. J Am Coll Cardiol Heart Fail 2018;6(9):757–67.

40. Kurozumi Y, Oishi S, Sugano Y, et al. Possible associations between palliative care conferences and positive outcomes when performing palliative care for patients with end-stage heart failure: a nationwide cross-sectional questionnaire survey. Heart Vessels 2019;34(3):452–61.

41. Cross SH, Kamal AH, Taylor DH Jr, et al. Hospice use among patients with heart failure. Card Fail Rev 2019;5(2):93–8.

Moving?

Make sure your subscription moves with you!

To notify us of your new address, find your **Clinics Account Number** (located on your mailing label above your name), and contact customer service at:

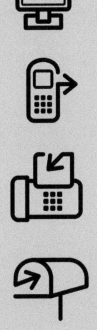

Email: journalscustomerservice-usa@elsevier.com

800-654-2452 (subscribers in the U.S. & Canada)
314-447-8871 (subscribers outside of the U.S. & Canada)

Fax number: 314-447-8029

Elsevier Health Sciences Division
Subscription Customer Service
3251 Riverport Lane
Maryland Heights, MO 63043

ELSEVIER

Printed and bound by CPI Group (UK) Ltd, Croydon, CR0 4YY

03/10/2024

01040307-0009